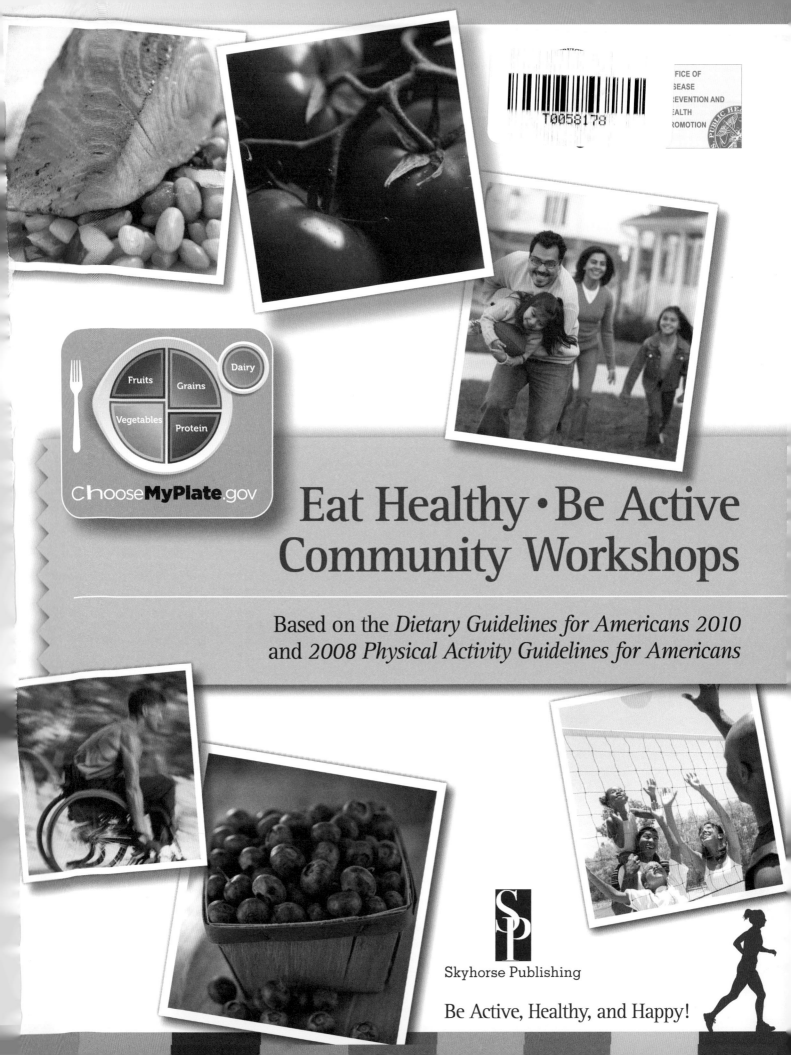

ChooseMyPlate.gov

Eat Healthy • Be Active Community Workshops

Based on the *Dietary Guidelines for Americans 2010* and *2008 Physical Activity Guidelines for Americans*

Skyhorse Publishing

Be Active, Healthy, and Happy!

Skyhorse Publishing books may be purchased in bulk at special discounts for sales promotion, corporate gifts, fund-raising, or educational purposes. Special editions can also be created to specifications. For details, contact the Special Sales Department, Skyhorse Publishing, 307 West 36th Street, 11th Floor, New York, NY 10018 or info@skyhorsepublishing.com.

Skyhorse® and Skyhorse Publishing® are registered trademarks of Skyhorse Publishing, Inc.®, a Delaware corporation.

Visit our website at www.skyhorsepublishing.com.

10 9 8 7 6 5 4 3 2 1

Library of Congress Cataloging-in-Publication Data is available on file.

Cover design by US Department of Health and Human Services

ISBN: 978-1-5107-2611-6
Ebook ISBN: 978-1-5107-2623-9

Printed in China

Eat Healthy ● Be Active Community Workshop Series

Contents

Eating and physical activity patterns that are focused on consuming fewer calories, making informed food choices, and being physically active can help people attain and maintain a healthy weight, reduce their risk of chronic disease, and promote overall health.
—Dietary Guidelines for Americans, 2010,
Executive Summary

The *Dietary Guidelines for Americans, 2010* and the *2008 Physical Activity Guidelines for Americans* provide science-based advice to promote health and reduce obesity and risk for major chronic diseases. Together, these two important publications provide guidance on the importance of being physically active and selecting nutritious foods for living a long and healthy life.

The *Dietary Guidelines for Americans* provide advice for making food choices that promote good health and a healthy weight and help prevent disease. The two main themes of these guidelines are balancing calories to manage body weight and focusing on foods and beverages that are high in nutrients (while controlling calorie and sodium intake). They encourage Americans to eat more healthy foods like vegetables, fruits, whole grains, fat-free and low-fat dairy products, and seafood and to consume less sodium, saturated and *trans* fats, added sugars, and refined grains. The guidelines also emphasize a flexible approach to eating patterns where individual tastes and food preferences are considered. There is also a stronger emphasis on balancing calorie intake with physical activity.

The *Physical Activity Guidelines for Americans* provide recommendations on the amount, types, and level of intensity of physical activity needed to achieve and maintain good health. These guidelines stress the importance of creating a physical activity plan that includes moderate- and/or vigorous-intensity aerobic activities and muscle-strengthening activities that are tailored to a person's specific interests, lifestyle, and goals.

The two guidelines go hand-in-hand and together provide important information for developing and maintaining a healthy lifestyle. They are the basis for the **Eat Healthy • Be Active Community Workshops.**

Community Leader's Role in Promoting Recommendations From the Guidelines and Implementing the Workshop Series

You play an active and important role in helping people attain and maintain a healthy weight, reduce their risk of chronic disease, and live a healthy lifestyle.

The Dietary Guidelines provide these selected consumer messages. More information about the messages can be found at http://www.ChooseMyPlate.gov.

Balancing Calories

✓ Enjoy your food, but eat less.

✓ Avoid oversized portions.

Foods to Increase

✓ Make half your plate fruits and vegetables.

✓ Make at least half your grains whole grains.

✓ Switch to fat-free or low-fat (1%) milk.

Foods to Decrease

✓ Compare sodium in foods like soup, bread, and frozen meals—and choose foods with lower numbers.

✓ Drink water instead of sugary drinks.

Healthy eating and physical activity work hand in hand to help us live healthier lives. The Physical Activity Guidelines recommend that adults be physically active for at least 2 hours and 30 minutes each week—children need 60 minutes each day.

✓ You can stay physically active by doing activities such as walking, dancing, bicycling, or gardening and by reducing the amount of time you spend sitting.

The Eat Healthy • Be Active Community Workshop Series builds on these concepts by providing detailed tips for how to put these recommended behaviors into practice. The workshops are designed to move participants from the "thinking" phase to taking desired health actions.

The workshops and corresponding materials are suitable for all groups of adults, including busy people with limited time and those with low health literacy. Health literacy is the degree to which people have the capacity to find, understand, and use basic health information. The U.S. Department of Health and Human Services (HHS) is committed to making the information from the Dietary Guidelines and Physical Activity Guidelines accessible to the majority of the U.S. adult population. The corresponding *Eat Healthy Your Way* handouts, included in the workshop series, were specifically developed and tested to provide information to help people of varying literacy levels make appropriate health and food selection decisions. In addition, the workshop series includes other handouts suitable for broader audiences, video vignettes, live demonstrations, and a list of helpful resources.

This information is packaged in six easy to conduct, interactive workshops. Each workshop contains learning objectives, icebreaker activities, talking points, instructions for stretch breaks, and hands-on learning activities, and provides opportunities to implement new practices that will lead to lasting lifestyle changes. The series includes:

1   **Enjoy Healthy Food That Tastes Great**

2   **Quick, Healthy Meals and Snacks**

3   **Eating Healthy on a Budget**

4   **Tips for Losing Weight and Keeping It Off**

5   **Making Healthy Eating Part of Your Total Lifestyle**

6   **Physical Activity Is Key to Living Well**

Optimally, the workshops can be offered in full as a series of six, or you can select the particular workshop(s) that would best fit the needs of your audience. For example, consider sharing "Tips for Losing Weight and Keeping It Off" with a group fitness class or offering "Enjoy Healthy Food That Tastes Great" to an existing community cooking class.

Your help is needed to find the best places in which to present the workshops to adults in your community who could benefit the most from learning more about eating healthfully and becoming more physically active. In addition to offering these workshops to community members, continue to assess the environment where you work and live to make sure that healthy lifestyle choices are easy, accessible, and desirable for all.

Please consider:

- Providing workshops to community groups with whom you are already working.

- Offering workshops to other groups within the community that would benefit from diet and physical activity recommendations, such as senior centers, PTAs, places of worship, exercise and recreation classes, etc.

- Helping to promote quarterly consumer messages. (http://www.ChooseMyPlate.gov/Partnerships/index.aspx)

- Planning events in your community that encourage physical activity and good health, such as fun runs, walks, contests, and challenges.

- Serving nutritious and healthy foods when refreshments are offered at events and programs.

- Incorporating stretch and movement breaks during events and programs.

- Recommending that local employers provide a work environment that encourages employees to be active and eat well.

- Modeling behaviors consistent with the recommendations for diet and physical activity.

Tips for Workshop Facilitators

- Prior to the workshop, make sure you have read and reviewed the entire workshop (until you are comfortable talking about the material) and gathered the materials that you will need (copies of handouts, healthy prizes, food ingredients, etc.). If you are teaching all of the workshops, see the suggested list of supplies (on the next page) so you can pull together everything you will need all at once. You may want to arrive 30 minutes ahead of time to prepare and make sure you have everything in place.

- When using talking points, be prepared to expand on the recommendations, give examples, and answer questions as they come up.

- A stretch break related to nutrition and physical activity (and included to promote a less sedentary way of living) is a component of each workshop. For Workshop 6, which includes a longer period of demonstration and physical activity, you may want to suggest to participants that they wear comfortable clothing. Workshop activities include games, demonstrations, and exercises designed to give participants a chance for hands-on learning.

- A workshop evaluation is provided for participants to complete at the end of each workshop. This information may be useful to share with local organization leaders/potential partners why it is important to provide support for the workshops.

- A reproducible *Certificate of Completion* has been included in the Appendix. This can be used to acknowledge participants for successful completion of the workshop series.

List of Supplies That May Be Needed

Nonfood items

- ❑ Crayons
- ❑ Markers
- ❑ Toothpicks
- ❑ Measuring cup
- ❑ Serving plate/tray
- ❑ Tablespoon and teaspoon (measuring spoons)
- ❑ Vegetable peeler
- ❑ Knife
- ❑ Cutting board
- ❑ Slow cooker
- ❑ Large serving bowl
- ❑ Can opener
- ❑ Disposable small and large plates, bowls, and spoons (for participants)
- ❑ Napkins
- ❑ Sales circulars from local grocery stores (one for every 2–3 participants)
- ❑ Nutrition facts labels from a variety of packaged foods (one for every 2–3 participants)
- ❑ Menus from local restaurants (American, Mexican, Chinese, Italian, deli, etc.)
- ❑ Healthy prizes: fruit, water bottle, jump rope, etc.
- ❑ Resistance bands of modest tension (or the soup cans listed below are fine)—you will need 1 band or 2 soup cans for each person

Food items

- ❑ 1 cup sugar
- ❑ 12-ounce can of sugar-sweetened soda
- ❑ Approximately 1 tablespoon each of a few of the following: thyme, basil, oregano, rosemary, garlic powder, onion powder, chili powder, cumin, low-sodium taco seasoning, low-sodium Italian seasoning, etc.
- ❑ 1 cup olive oil
- ❑ Salt-free pretzels (enough to serve each participant 3–4)
- ❑ Store-brand canned fruit in unsweetened juice (enough for each participant to have a few bites of the fruit)
- ❑ Name-brand canned fruit in unsweetened juice (enough for each participant to have a few bites of the fruit)
- ❑ Large pepper (green, red, or yellow)
- ❑ Large onion
- ❑ Large zucchini
- ❑ 2 large carrots
- ❑ 2 cloves garlic
- ❑ 1½ teaspoons oregano
- ❑ 1 pound boneless/skinless chicken breasts (approximately 4) or lean ground beef or ground turkey
- ❑ 14½-ounce can of no-salt-added tomatoes
- ❑ Assorted fruits and vegetables (including some that may be unfamiliar to the population you are teaching), cut up for tasting
- ❑ 2 soup cans for each workshop participant (unless you have resistance bands)
- ❑ Assorted whole grain products (may need to be cut up or cooked prior to tasting, depending on foods selected)

Workshop 1

Enjoy Healthy Food That Tastes Great

Eat Healthy ● *Be Active*
Community Workshops

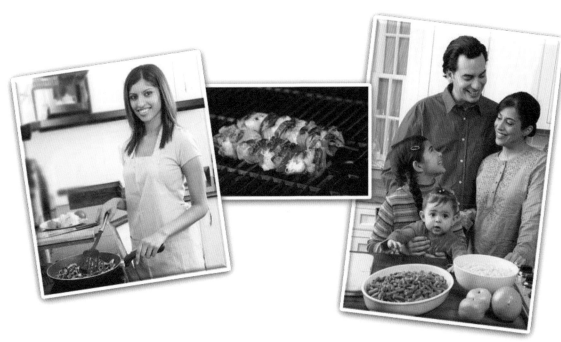

OFFICE OF
DISEASE
PREVENTION AND
HEALTH
PROMOTION

Instructor Guide

Before Workshop Begins

- Thoroughly read entire workshop and become familiar with the lesson plan.
- Choose an activity to do, and gather materials needed for the icebreaker and the chosen activity.
  - *Icebreaker:* large and small disposable plates, salt-free pretzels, olive oil, a selection of spices (hint: consider buying spices from a food co-op where you can buy small amounts for less money), and a plate/tray for the spices
  - *Activity 1:* paper plates, crayons/markers/etc. for each person
  - *Activity 2:* sugar, can of soda, plate, teaspoon
- Photocopy handouts (one per participant):
  1. Enjoy Healthy Food That Tastes Great (2 pages)
  2. Find Someone Who... (1 page)
  3. Tips for Healthier Choices (2 pages)
  4. Reduce Your Sodium (Salt) Intake (1 page)
  5. Modifying a Recipe/Recipe Makeover (2 pages)
  6. MyPlate/10 Tips to a Great Plate (2 pages)
  7. Workshop Evaluation (1 page)

Workshop Outline

The workshop should last ~1 hour, including activities.

- Icebreaker activity (5 minutes)—do this while people are coming into the workshop
- Introduction (5 minutes)
  - Explain the purpose of the workshop
  - Review the Learning Objectives
- **Objective 1:** Learn about small changes you can make to choose healthier fats, less salt, and less added sugars (5–10 minutes)
  - Review handout: *Enjoy Healthy Food That Tastes Great*
- Video: *Healthy Can Be Tasty* (2–3 minutes)

- Stretch Break (5 minutes)
  - Review handout: *Find Someone Who. . .*
- **Objective 2:** Learn about food substitutions and using spices, herbs, and salt-free seasonings that will give you new ways to eat healthfully (5–10 minutes)
  - Review handout: *Tips for Healthier Choices*
  - Review handout: *Reduce Your Sodium (Salt) Intake*
- Activity (5–10 minutes). *Note:* Choose ahead of time and gather supplies. If doing Activity 1, review *10 Tips to a Great Plate* during this time
- **Objective 3:** Learn ideas for recipe modifications and cooking techniques to reduce calories, solid fats (saturated and *trans* fat), sodium, or added sugars (5–10 minutes)
  - Review handout: *Modifying a Recipe/Recipe Makeover* (at-home activity)
- Increasing Physical Activity (1–2 minutes)
- Review handout *MyPlate* and how to use *10 Tips to a Great Plate* (2 minutes)
- Wrap-up/Q&A (5 minutes)
  - Reminders of things to try at home:
    - Modify a recipe to make it lower in solid fats (saturated and *trans* fat), sodium, or added sugars
    - Reduce amount of screen time and increase physical activity
- Ask participants to complete the evaluation form (5 minutes)

Workshop Lesson Plan

Icebreaker Activity—Taste Testing (5 minutes)

Spices/Herbs/Seasoning Taste Test: Select 2–3 spices, such as thyme, basil, oregano, rosemary, garlic powder, onion powder, chili powder, low-sodium taco seasoning, cumin, curry, coriander, salt-free seasoning mixes, etc. As people come into the workshop, offer them a salt-free pretzel to dip in a small amount of olive oil and then in a spice. See how they like the taste and whether they can name the spice/seasoning.

Supplies necessary: Large and small disposable plates, salt-free pretzels, olive oil, a selection of spices (hint: consider buying spices from a food co-op where you can buy small amounts for less money), and a plate/tray for the spices.

Talking Points—Purpose of the Workshop (2–3 minutes)

- Today's workshop and handouts will give you tips for making meals that are both healthy and taste great.

- This workshop is based on the *Dietary Guidelines for Americans, 2010* and the *2008 Physical Activity Guidelines for Americans*. The Dietary Guidelines provide science-based advice for making food choices that promote good health and a healthy weight and help prevent disease. The Physical Activity Guidelines provide recommendations on the amount, types, and level of intensity of physical activity needed to achieve and maintain good health.

- The Dietary Guidelines provide these selected consumer messages. More information about the messages can be found at http://www.ChooseMyPlate.gov/.
  - *Balancing Calories*
    - ✓ Enjoy your food, but eat less.
    - ✓ Avoid oversized portions.
  - *Foods to Increase*
    - ✓ Make half your plate fruits and vegetables.
    - ✓ Make at least half your grains whole grains.
    - ✓ Switch to fat-free or low-fat (1%) milk.

- *Foods to Decrease*

  ✓ Compare sodium in foods like soup, bread, and frozen meals—and choose foods with lower numbers.

  ✓ Drink water instead of sugary drinks.

- Healthy eating and physical activity work hand in hand to help us live healthier lives. The Physical Activity Guidelines recommend that adults be physically active for at least 2 hours and 30 minutes each week—children need 60 minutes each day.

  ✓ You can stay physically active by doing activities such as walking, dancing, bicycling, or gardening and by reducing the amount of time you spend sitting.

Talking Points—Learning Objectives (2–3 minutes)

1. Learn about small changes you can make to choose healthier fats, less salt, and less added sugars.

2. Learn about food substitutions and using spices, herbs, and salt-free seasonings that will give you new ways to eat healthfully.

3. Learn ideas for recipe modifications and cooking techniques to reduce calories, solid fats (saturated and *trans* fat), sodium, or added sugars.

Talking Points—Handout: Enjoy Healthy Food That Tastes Great (5–10 minutes)

Small Changes Can Make a Large Difference

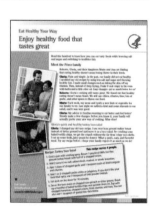

- Select leaner cuts of ground beef (90% lean or higher), turkey breast, or chicken breast.

- Compare sodium in foods like soup, bread, and frozen meals—and choose foods with lower numbers.

- Limit your purchase of processed meats, which tend to be high in sodium.

- Try seafood instead of meat and poultry. You should aim to eat 8 ounces of seafood per week. See Appendix 11 in the *Dietary Guidelines for Americans* for information on mercury content of fish.

- Choose whole-grain cereals that don't have frosting or added sugars; add flavor to hot whole-grain cereals with raisins, vanilla, and/or cinnamon.

- Make half your plate fruits and vegetables (especially nutrient-packed ones that are red, orange, and green, as well as beans and peas).

  - Choose frozen vegetables without sauces and canned vegetables that are labeled as reduced sodium or no-salt-added.

  - In addition to fresh fruits, use canned, frozen, and dried fruits. Look for unsweetened fruit or fruit canned in 100% juice.

- Choose water, fat-free or low-fat milk, 100% fruit juice, or unsweetened tea or coffee as drinks rather than regular soda, sports drinks, energy drinks, fruit drinks, and other sugar-sweetened drinks.

- Instead of a big dessert, try a piece of fresh fruit or a frozen fruit bar, or split a smaller dessert with a friend.

Video: Healthy Can Be Tasty (2–3 minutes)

Stretch Break—Handout: Find Someone Who. . . (5 minutes)

"Find Someone Who . . .": This bingo-like game reinforces the winning combination of a healthy diet and physical activity, and allows participants to get to know one another. Pass out the game sheet and ask participants to walk around the room and talk to one another to learn which healthy lifestyle activities each person enjoys. Participants then sign their names in the boxes for the activities they do. Depending on the size of the group, set a limit on how many boxes the same person can sign on a participant's game sheet (usually just two). Award a healthy prize (fruit, water bottle, 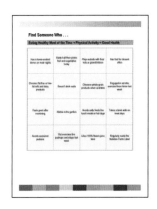 jump rope, etc.) to the first person to get a complete row signed. To keep the game going, ask participants to try and complete two rows, a "T" pattern, or even the whole grid. It's helpful to have several prizes on hand to reward winners.

Supplies necessary: *Find Someone Who . . .* handout for each participant, healthy prize items

Talking Points—Handout: Tips for Healthier Choices (5 minutes)

The Dietary Guidelines recommend eating less of several foods and food components. By cutting back on these foods, you can reduce your intake of sodium, cholesterol, solid fats (saturated and *trans* fat), added sugars, and refined grains.

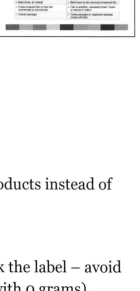

- Reduce daily **sodium** intake to less than 2,300 mg/day (see note below for special populations to reduce to less than 1,500 mg/day).

    ✓ *Here's how:* Choose low-sodium or no-salt-added canned goods.

- Consume less than 300 mg per day of dietary **cholesterol.**

    ✓ *Here's how:* Try using egg substitutes for whole eggs.

- Consume less than 10% of calories from **saturated fats.**

    ✓ *Here's how:* Choose lean meats and fat-free or low-fat dairy products instead of whole or 2% dairy foods.

- Keep ***trans* fatty acid** consumption as low as possible.

    ✓ *Here's how:* Limit foods with partially hydrogenated oils (check the label – avoid foods with any *trans* fat and check the ingredient list of foods with 0 grams).

- Reduce the intake of calories from **added sugars.**

    ✓ *Here's how:* Choose foods prepared with little or no added sugars.

- Limit **refined grains.**

    ✓ *Here's how:* Choose whole-grain bread, brown rice, whole-wheat flour, or whole-grain pasta.

Talking Points—Handout: Reduce Your Sodium (Salt) Intake (5 minutes)

- Too much sodium can be bad for your health. It can increase your blood pressure and your risk for a heart attack and stroke.

- The majority of sodium we consume is in processed and restaurant foods.

- The average sodium intake for Americans over age 2 is approximately **3,400 mg** per day.

- The Dietary Guidelines recommend reducing sodium intake to less than **2,300 mg** of sodium per day.

- *Note:* Children and those in the following population groups should reduce intake to **1,500 mg** of sodium per day:

  - Those who are 51 years of age or older.

  - Those who are African American.

  - Those who have high blood pressure.

  - Those who have diabetes.

  - Those who have chronic kidney disease.

Activity—Choose One Ahead of Time (5–10 minutes)

1. **"MyPlate" Drawing:** Give each participant a paper plate and ask the group to draw pictures of foods that make up a healthy plate. Remind them to design a plate that is half fruits and vegetables and features whole grains, lean protein, low-fat dairy products, and foods that are low in sodium. Cover the *10 Tips to a Great Plate* handout immediately prior to this activity instead of waiting to the end of the workshop. Ask each participant to show his or her plate and describe his or her proposed meal to the group.

   Supplies necessary: paper plates, crayons/markers/etc. for each person

2. **Demonstration: How much sugar is in a soda?** Ask participants to guess how many teaspoons are in a can of soda before you start this activity. Ask for a volunteer to help you with this demonstration. Ask the volunteer to spoon out 10 teaspoons of sugar onto a plate in front of a can of regular soda. Then tell participants that this is about the amount of sugar in one can of soda. Ask participants: If you drank a 12-ounce regular soda every day for a year, how much sugar would that be? The answer is 30 pounds of sugar! Let them know that a person could lose up to 15 pounds in a year by switching from 1 can of regular soda per day (150 calories) to water or another calorie-free drink.

   Supplies necessary: sugar, can of soda, plate, teaspoon

Talking Points—Handout: Modifying a Recipe/Recipe Makeover (5–10 minutes)

There are simple changes you can make when cooking to reduce calories, solid fats (saturated and *trans* fat), sodium (salt), or added sugars. Here are some general tips to make your meals healthier.

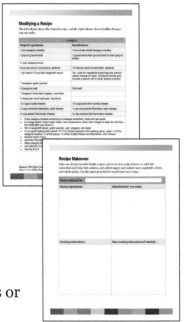

- Cook with low-fat methods such as baking, broiling, boiling, or microwaving, rather than frying.

- Season foods with herbs, spices, lime or lemon juice, and vinegar rather than salt.

- Use oils and spray oils instead of solid fats like butter and margarine.

- Increase the amount of vegetables and/or fruit in a recipe— remember, you want to fill half of your plate with vegetables or fruits.

- Take the skin off chicken and turkey pieces before cooking them.

- Reduce the amount of sugar by one-quarter to one-third. For example, if a recipe calls for 1 cup, use 2/3 cup. To enhance the flavor when sugar is reduced, add vanilla, cinnamon, or nutmeg.

Talking Points—Increasing Physical Activity (1-2 minutes)

- The *Physical Activity Guidelines for Americans* recommend that everyone engage in regular physical activity for health benefits.

- Here are the recommendations for adults:

	Moderate Activity	Vigorous Activity
Types of Activity	Walking briskly, biking on flat ground, line dancing, gardening	Jumping rope, basketball, soccer, swimming laps, aerobic dance
Amount	If you choose activities at a **moderate** level, do at least **2 hours and 30 minutes a week**	If you choose activities at a **vigorous** level, do at least **1 hour and 15 minutes a week**

- You can combine moderate and vigorous activities. In general, 1 minute of vigorous activity is equal to 2 minutes of moderate activity.

- Children need **60 minutes of physical activity each day.**

- **TODAY'S TIP:** Limit screen time.
  - ✓ Limit the amount of time you spend watching TV or other media such as video games. This is especially important for children and adolescents.
  - ✓ Use the time you watch TV to be physically active in front of the TV.
- Consider signing up for the Presidential Active Lifestyle Award (PALA+) to help you track your physical activity and take small steps to improve your eating habits.
- If you are active for 30 minutes a day, 5 days a week for 6 out of 8 weeks, and choose one healthy eating goal each week to work toward, you'll be awarded the PALA+ and receive Presidential recognition! (See http://www.presidentschallenge.org). See handout in Appendix for more information.

Talking Points—Handouts: MyPlate and 10 Tips (2 minutes)

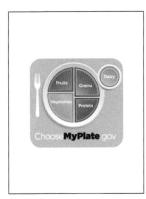
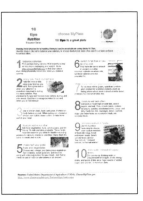

Talking Points—Wrap-up/Q&A (5 minutes)

Things to Try at Home
- Modify a recipe to make it lower in solid fats (saturated and *trans* fat), sodium, or added sugars.
- Reduce amount of screen time and increase physical activity.

Complete Evaluation Form (5 minutes)

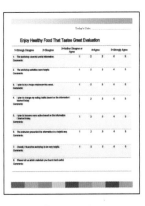

Workshop 1 ● Handouts

Eat Healthy Your Way

Enjoy healthy food that tastes great

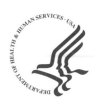

Read this handout to learn how you can eat tasty foods while lowering salt and sugar and switching to healthier fats.

Meet the Pérez family

Roberto, Gloria, and their daughters Marta and Ana are finding that eating healthy doesn't mean losing flavor in their foods.

Gloria: Plain and simple—in the past, our family did not eat healthy. I modified my old recipes by using less salt and sugar and choosing healthy fats. I made small changes such as taking the skin off my chicken. Then, instead of deep-frying, I bake it real crispy in the oven with herbs and a little olive oil. Easy changes—yet so much better for us!

Roberto: Gloria's cooking still tastes great. We found out that healthy eating doesn't mean bland. We still use chiles, cilantro, lime, lots of garlic, and other spices to flavor our food.

Marta: Each week, my mom and I pick a new fruit or vegetable for our family to try. Last night we added a kiwi and some almonds to our salad, and it was very good.

Gloria: My advice to families wanting to eat better and feel better? Slowly make a few changes. Before you know it, your family will actually prefer your new way of cooking. Mine does!

Gloria's quick and healthy turkey taco salad

Gloria: I changed my old taco recipe. I use very lean ground turkey breast instead of fattier ground beef and serve it as a taco salad. By crushing some baked tortilla chips, we get the crunch without the fat from crispy taco shells. I cut up some fresh, juicy pears for dessert. What a quick, easy, and flavorful meal. Try my recipe below—I hope your family enjoys it as much as we do!

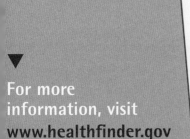

Recipe: Turkey Taco Salad

This recipe serves 4 people.

1. Coat a pan with cooking spray. Brown 1 pound of 99% fat-free ground turkey breast with half of a chopped onion.
2. Add 2 cans of no-salt-added diced, crushed, or whole tomatoes.
3. Add 1 clove of chopped garlic and 1 teaspoon each of dried oregano and cilantro.
4. Add 1 or 2 chopped ancho chiles or jalapenos. If you don't like your food that spicy, use 2 teaspoons of chili powder instead.
5. Let cook on the stove for 10 minutes.
6. Serve the taco meat on chopped raw spinach or other greens. Break up a handful of baked tortilla chips and sprinkle them on. Top with chopped tomatoes, chopped onions, fresh cilantro, and lime. You can also add 1 teaspoon of grated low-fat cheese.

For more information, visit www.healthfinder.gov

(turn over please)

Small changes can make a large difference

All the flavor—with healthy fats, less salt, and less sugar!

Check off the tips you will try.

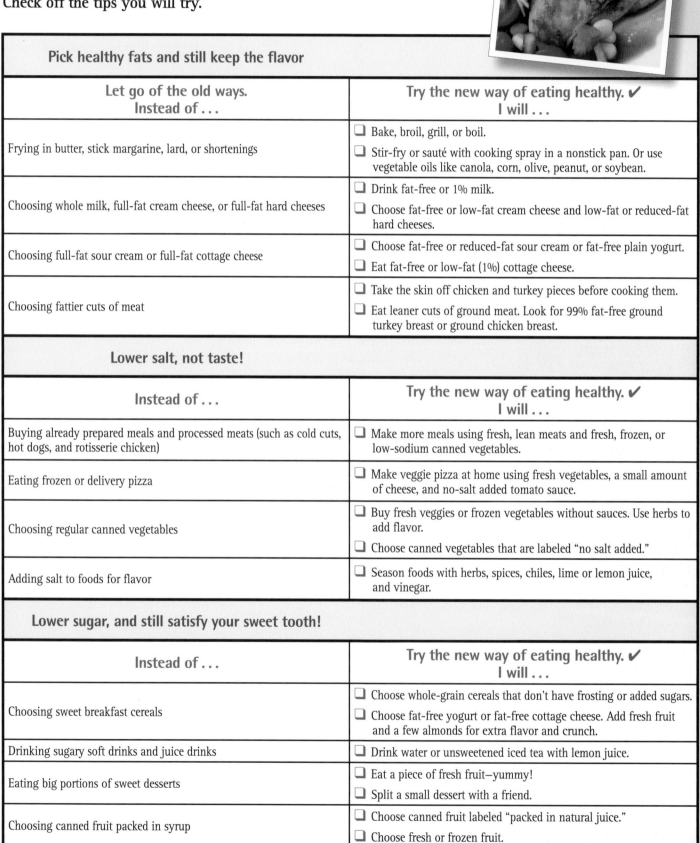

Pick healthy fats and still keep the flavor	
Let go of the old ways. **Instead of . . .**	**Try the new way of eating healthy. ✔** **I will . . .**
Frying in butter, stick margarine, lard, or shortenings	❑ Bake, broil, grill, or boil. ❑ Stir-fry or sauté with cooking spray in a nonstick pan. Or use vegetable oils like canola, corn, olive, peanut, or soybean.
Choosing whole milk, full-fat cream cheese, or full-fat hard cheeses	❑ Drink fat-free or 1% milk. ❑ Choose fat-free or low-fat cream cheese and low-fat or reduced-fat hard cheeses.
Choosing full-fat sour cream or full-fat cottage cheese	❑ Choose fat-free or reduced-fat sour cream or fat-free plain yogurt. ❑ Eat fat-free or low-fat (1%) cottage cheese.
Choosing fattier cuts of meat	❑ Take the skin off chicken and turkey pieces before cooking them. ❑ Eat leaner cuts of ground meat. Look for 99% fat-free ground turkey breast or ground chicken breast.

Lower salt, not taste!	
Instead of . . .	**Try the new way of eating healthy. ✔** **I will . . .**
Buying already prepared meals and processed meats (such as cold cuts, hot dogs, and rotisserie chicken)	❑ Make more meals using fresh, lean meats and fresh, frozen, or low-sodium canned vegetables.
Eating frozen or delivery pizza	❑ Make veggie pizza at home using fresh vegetables, a small amount of cheese, and no-salt added tomato sauce.
Choosing regular canned vegetables	❑ Buy fresh veggies or frozen vegetables without sauces. Use herbs to add flavor. ❑ Choose canned vegetables that are labeled "no salt added."
Adding salt to foods for flavor	❑ Season foods with herbs, spices, chiles, lime or lemon juice, and vinegar.

Lower sugar, and still satisfy your sweet tooth!	
Instead of . . .	**Try the new way of eating healthy. ✔** **I will . . .**
Choosing sweet breakfast cereals	❑ Choose whole-grain cereals that don't have frosting or added sugars. ❑ Choose fat-free yogurt or fat-free cottage cheese. Add fresh fruit and a few almonds for extra flavor and crunch.
Drinking sugary soft drinks and juice drinks	❑ Drink water or unsweetened iced tea with lemon juice.
Eating big portions of sweet desserts	❑ Eat a piece of fresh fruit—yummy! ❑ Split a small dessert with a friend.
Choosing canned fruit packed in syrup	❑ Choose canned fruit labeled "packed in natural juice." ❑ Choose fresh or frozen fruit.

ODPHP Publication No. U0051

January 2011

Find Someone Who . . .

Eating Healthy Most of the Time + Physical Activity = Good Health

Has a home-cooked dinner on most nights	Made half their plates fruit and vegetables today	Plays outside with their kids or grandchildren	Has fruit for dessert often
Chooses fat-free or low-fat milk and dairy products	Doesn't drink soda	Chooses whole-grain products when available	Engaged in aerobic exercise three times last week
Feels good after exercising	Works in the garden	Avoids salty foods like lunch meats or hot dogs	Takes a brisk walk on most days
Avoids oversized portions	Did exercises like pushups and situps last week	Likes 100% frozen juice bars	Regularly reads the Nutrition Facts Label

Tips for Healthier Choices

These alternatives provide new ideas for old favorites. Don't forget to check food labels to compare calories, solid fats (saturated and *trans* fat), and sodium in products.

If you usually buy:	Try these:
Milk and Milk Products	
• Whole milk (regular, evaporated, or sweetened condensed)	• Fat-free (skim), low-fat (1%) milk, evaporated milk, or sweetened condensed milk
• Ice cream	• Sorbet and ices, sherbet, or low-fat or fat-free frozen yogurt
• Sour cream	• Plain fat-free or low-fat Greek yogurt or fat-free sour cream
• Cream cheese	• Neufchatel "light" cream cheese or fat-free cream cheese
• Cheese (cheddar, Swiss, Monterey Jack, American, mozzarella, etc.)	• Reduced-calorie or fat-free cheese, part-skim, low-calorie processed cheeses, etc.
• Regular (4%) cottage cheese	• Fat-free or low-fat (1%) cottage cheese
• Whole-milk ricotta cheese	• Part-skim milk ricotta cheese
• Coffee cream (½ and ½) or nondairy creamer	• Low-fat (1%) or nonfat dry milk powder
Cereals, Grains, and Pastas	
• Pasta with white sauce (Alfredo)	• Whole grain pasta with red sauce (marinara)
• Pasta with cheese sauce	• Whole grain pasta with vegetables (primavera)
• White rice or pasta	• Brown rice or whole grain pasta
Meats, Fish, and Poultry	
• Cold cuts or lunch meats (bologna, salami, liverwurst, etc.)	• Low-fat/reduced sodium cold cuts (turkey, chicken)
• Bacon or sausage	• Canadian bacon or lean ham
• Regular ground beef	• Extra-lean ground beef or lean ground turkey
• Beef chuck, rib, brisket	• Beef round or loin (trimmed of external fat)
• Frozen breaded fish or fried fish (homemade or commercial)	• Fish or shellfish, unbreaded (fresh, frozen, or canned in water)
• Chorizo sausage	• Turkey sausage or vegetarian sausage (made with tofu)

If you usually buy:	Try these:
Baked Goods	
• Croissants or brioches	• Whole grain rolls
• Doughnuts, sweet rolls, muffins, scones, or pastries	• Whole grain English muffins, bagels, reduced-fat or fat-free muffins or scones
• Party crackers or cookies	• Saltine or soda crackers, pretzels, whole grain crackers (choose lower in sodium), graham crackers, ginger snaps, or fig bars
• Frosted cake or pound cake	• Angel food cake or gingerbread
Fats, Oils, and Salad Dressings	
• Regular margarine or butter	• Light margarines or olive oil
• Regular mayonnaise	• Mustard or fat-free or reduced-fat mayonnaise
• Regular salad dressing	• Fat-free or reduced-fat salad dressings, lemon juice, or wine vinegar
• Oils, shortening, or lard for pan cooking	• Nonstick cooking spray for stir-frying or sautéing
Miscellaneous	
• Canned cream soups	• Canned broth-based soups (low sodium)
• Gravy (homemade with fat and/or milk)	• Gravy mixes made with water or homemade with the fat skimmed off and fat-free milk

Reduce Your Sodium (Salt) Intake

- Read the Nutrition Facts Labels to choose foods lower in sodium.

- When purchasing canned foods, select those labeled as "reduced sodium," "low sodium," or "no salt added." Rinse regular canned foods to remove some sodium.

- Gradually reduce the amount of sodium in your foods. Your taste for salt will change over time.

- Consume more fresh food and few processed foods that are high in sodium.

- Eat more home-prepared foods, where you have more control over sodium, and use little or no salt or salt-containing seasonings when cooking or eating foods.

- When eating at restaurants, ask that salt not be added to your food or order lower sodium options, if available.

Tips for Using Herbs and Spices (Instead of Salt)	
Basil:	Use in soups, salads, vegetables, fish, and meats.
Cinnamon:	Use in salads, vegetables, breads, and snacks.
Chili Powder:	Use in soups, salads, vegetables, and fish.
Cloves:	Use in soups, salads, and vegetables.
Dill Weed and Dill Seed:	Use in fish, soups, salads, and vegetables.
Ginger:	Use in soups, salads, vegetables, and meats.
Garlic:	Use in soups, vegetables, meats, and chicken.
Marjoram:	Use in soups, salads, vegetables, beef, fish, and chicken.
Nutmeg:	Use in vegetables, meats, and snacks.
Oregano:	Use in soups, salads, vegetables, meats, and chicken.
Parsley:	Use in salads, vegetables, fish, and meats.
Rosemary:	Use in salads, vegetables, fish, and meats.
Sage:	Use in soups, salads, vegetables, meats, and chicken.
Thyme:	Use in salads, vegetables, fish, and chicken.

Note: To start, use small amounts of these herbs and spices to see whether you like them.

Source: Dietary Guidelines for Americans, *A Healthier You, Part III.*
http://www.health.gov/dietaryguidelines/dga2005/healthieryou/contents.htm

Modifying a Recipe

The left column shows the original recipe, and the right column shows healthy changes you can make.

Lasagna	
Original Ingredients:	**Substitutions:**
1 box lasagna noodles	1 box whole-wheat lasagna noodles
1 pound ground beef	1 pound extra-lean ground beef or lean ground turkey
½ cup chopped onion	
8 ounces sliced mushrooms, optional	12 ounces sliced mushrooms, optional
1 jar (about 16 ounces) spaghetti sauce	Tip: Look for vegetable-based sauces without added cheese or meat. Compare brands and choose a sauce with a lower sodium content.
1 teaspoon garlic powder	
½ teaspoon salt	Omit salt
1 teaspoon dried leaf oregano, crumbled	
½ teaspoon dried leaf basil, crumbled	
1½ cups ricotta cheese	1½ cups part-skim ricotta cheese
2 cups shredded Monterey Jack cheese	1 cup reduced-fat Monterey Jack cheese
¾ cup grated Parmesan cheese	½ cup reduced-fat Parmesan cheese

- Cook lasagna noodles according to package directions; drain and set aside.
- In a large skillet, brown beef, onion, and mushrooms. *Note:* Don't forget to drain the fat from the meat after you brown it.
- Stir in spaghetti sauce, garlic powder, salt, oregano, and basil.
- In a 2-quart baking dish (about 11×7×2 inches) sprayed with cooking spray, layer ⅓ of the lasagna noodles, ⅓ of the sauce, ⅓ of the ricotta cheese and Monterey Jack cheese.
- Repeat layers twice.
- Sprinkle Parmesan cheese on top.
- Bake lasagna for 30 minutes or until thoroughly heated and bubbly in a 350°F oven.
- Let stand for 8 to 10 minutes before cutting and serving.
- Serves 6 to 8.

Source: *We Can!* Fun Family Recipes & Tips
http://www.nhlbi.nih.gov/health/public/heart/obesity/wecan/eat-right/fun-family-recipes.htm

Recipe Makeover

Take one of your favorite family recipes and revise it to make it lower in solid fats (saturated and *trans* fat), sodium, and added sugars and include more vegetables, fruits, and whole grains. Use the space provided to record your new recipe.

Recipe makeover for	
Recipe ingredients:	**Substitutions I can make:**
Cooking instructions:	**New cooking instructions (if needed):**

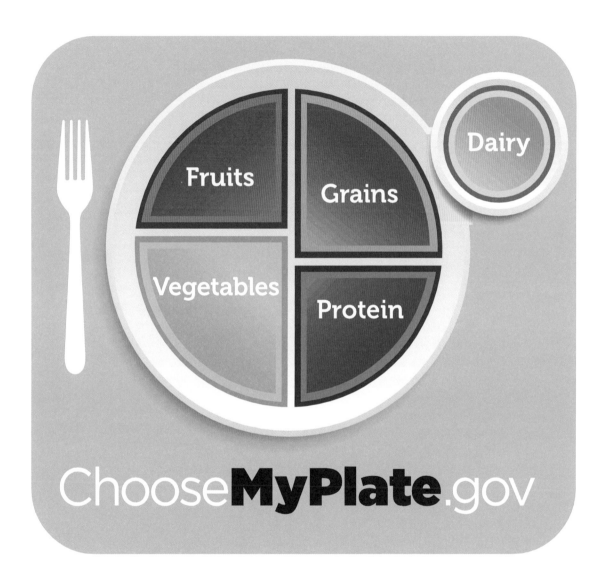

Fruits

Grains

Vegetables

Protein

Dairy

ChooseMyPlate.gov

10 tips
Nutrition Education Series

choose MyPlate
10 tips to a great plate

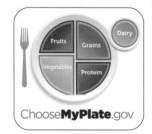

ChooseMyPlate.gov

Making food choices for a healthy lifestyle can be as simple as using these 10 Tips.
Use the ideas in this list to *balance your calories*, to choose foods to *eat more often*, and to cut back on foods to *eat less often*.

1 balance calories
Find out how many calories YOU need for a day as a first step in managing your weight. Go to www.ChooseMyPlate.gov to find your calorie level. Being physically active also helps you balance calories.

2 enjoy your food, but eat less
Take the time to fully enjoy your food as you eat it. Eating too fast or when your attention is elsewhere may lead to eating too many calories. Pay attention to hunger and fullness cues before, during, and after meals. Use them to recognize when to eat and when you've had enough.

3 avoid oversized portions
Use a smaller plate, bowl, and glass. Portion out foods before you eat. When eating out, choose a smaller size option, share a dish, or take home part of your meal.

4 foods to eat more often
Eat more vegetables, fruits, whole grains, and fat-free or 1% milk and dairy products. These foods have the nutrients you need for health—including potassium, calcium, vitamin D, and fiber. Make them the basis for meals and snacks.

5 make half your plate fruits and vegetables
Choose red, orange, and dark-green vegetables like tomatoes, sweet potatoes, and broccoli, along with other vegetables for your meals. Add fruit to meals as part of main or side dishes or as dessert.

6 switch to fat-free or low-fat (1%) milk
They have the same amount of calcium and other essential nutrients as whole milk, but fewer calories and less saturated fat.

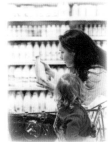

7 make half your grains whole grains
To eat more whole grains, substitute a whole-grain product for a refined product—such as eating whole-wheat bread instead of white bread or brown rice instead of white rice.

8 foods to eat less often
Cut back on foods high in solid fats, added sugars, and salt. They include cakes, cookies, ice cream, candies, sweetened drinks, pizza, and fatty meats like ribs, sausages, bacon, and hot dogs. Use these foods as occasional treats, not everyday foods.

9 compare sodium in foods
Use the Nutrition Facts label to choose lower sodium versions of foods like soup, bread, and frozen meals. Select canned foods labeled "low sodium," "reduced sodium," or "no salt added."

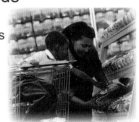

10 drink water instead of sugary drinks
Cut calories by drinking water or unsweetened beverages. Soda, energy drinks, and sports drinks are a major source of added sugar, and calories, in American diets.

USDA
United States
Department of Agriculture
Center for Nutrition
Policy and Promotion

Go to www.ChooseMyPlate.gov for more information.

DG TipSheet No. 1
June 2011
USDA is an equal opportunity provider and employer.

Enjoy Healthy Food That Tastes Great Evaluation

1=Strongly Disagree	2=Disagree	3=Neither Disagree or Agree	4=Agree	5=Strongly Agree

	1	2	3	4	5
1. The workshop covered useful information. Comments:	1	2	3	4	5
2. The workshop activities were helpful. Comments:	1	2	3	4	5
3. I plan to try a recipe makeover this week. Comments:	1	2	3	4	5
4. I plan to change my eating habits based on the information I learned today. Comments:	1	2	3	4	5
5. I plan to become more active based on the information I learned today. Comments:	1	2	3	4	5
6. The instructor presented the information in a helpful way. Comments:	1	2	3	4	5
7. Overall, I found the workshop to be very helpful. Comments:	1	2	3	4	5

8. Please tell us which materials you found most useful.
Comments:

Workshop 2

Quick, Healthy Meals and Snacks

Eat Healthy ● *Be Active*
Community Workshops

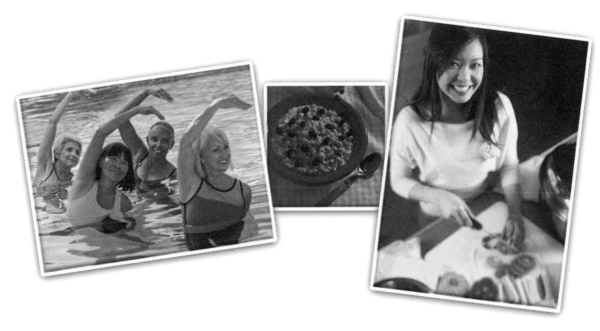

Instructor Guide

Before Workshop Begins

- Thoroughly read the entire workshop and become familiar with the lesson plan.

- Choose an activity to do, and gather materials needed for the icebreaker and the chosen activity.

  - *Icebreaker:* no supplies necessary

  - *Activity 1:* slow cooker, chopped green, red, or yellow peppers, onion, zucchini, carrots, 1 pound skinless chicken breasts or lean beef, 14½-oz can of no-salt-added diced tomatoes, 1½ teaspoons oregano, two cloves of garlic, minced, can opener

  - *Activity 2:* menus from local restaurants (including a range of ethnically diverse dishes), highlighters or pens to highlight or circle healthy options

Note about Activity 1: If you would like to serve the slow cooker meal at the workshop, you will need to cook the meal prior to class (the slow cooker will take several hours to complete). Or, you can demonstrate putting the ingredients into the slow cooker early in class and turn the slow cooker on high so that participants will be able to smell the food cooking. If demonstrating the slow cooker during class, you will need to chop the vegetables ahead of time (before class). Also, if you will be presenting the workshop in a location without a sink to wash your hands after placing the meat in the slow cooker, you can put the chicken/beef into a sealed plastic bag and then empty the bag into the slow cooker without touching the meat. See Appendix for additional information on food safety, as well as additional recipes.

- Photocopy handouts (one per participant):
  1. Quick, Healthy Meals and Snacks (2 pages)
  2. My Shopping List (1 page)
  3. Tips for Eating Out (1 page)
  4. Tips for Choosing Healthier Foods at Restaurants (2 pages)
  5. Slow Cooker Tips and Recipes (2 pages)
  6. MyPlate/10 Tips to Build a Healthy Meal (2 pages)
  7. Workshop Evaluation (1 page)

Workshop Outline

The workshop should last ~1 hour, including activities.

- Icebreaker activity (5 minutes)

- Introduction (5 minutes)

  – Explain the purpose of the workshop

  – Review the Learning Objectives

- **Objective 1:** Learn tips for preparing meals quickly and how to stock your pantry (5–10 minutes)

  – Review handout: *Quick, Healthy Meals and Snacks*

  – Review handout: *My Shopping List*

- Video: *Make It Fast, Make It Good* (2–3 minutes)

- Stretch Break (5 minutes)

- **Objective 2:** Learn how to make healthy selections when eating out (5–10 minutes)

  – Review handout: *Tips for Eating Out*

  – Review handout: *Tips for Choosing Healthier Foods at Restaurants*

- Activity (5–10 minutes). *Note:* If doing Activity 1, recommend doing it at the beginning of class as the icebreaker, so that the food cooks during the class

- **Objective 3:** Learn how to use a slow cooker to prepare easy, healthy meals (5–10 minutes)

  – Review handout: *Slow Cooker Tips and Recipes*

- Increasing Physical Activity (1–2 minutes)

- Review handout *MyPlate* and how to use *10 Tips to Build a Healthy Meal* (2 minutes)

- Wrap-up/Q&A (5 minutes)

  – Reminders of things to try at home:

    ▪ Next time you go to a restaurant, order a healthy dish using the tips for choosing items lower in calories, solid fats (saturated and *trans* fat), and sodium

    ▪ Increase the total amount of time you spend doing physical activity

- Ask participants to complete the evaluation form (5 minutes)

Workshop Lesson Plan

Icebreaker Activity (5 minutes)

Read the following questions out loud to participants. Ask them to raise their hands to indicate "frequently," "sometimes," or "almost never" in response to each question.

Are You an Effective Kitchen Manager?

	Frequently	Sometimes	Almost Never
How often do you plan meals in advance?			
How often do you prepare portions of a meal in advance?			
How often do you spend 30 minutes or less preparing a meal?			
How often do you use leftovers as the basis for another meal?			
If there are others in your household, how often do they help fix meals and clean up?			

After completing the questions, relay this information to participants: If you answered "frequently" to the questions, you probably manage your time very well. If you answered with "sometimes" or "almost never," don't throw in the dish towel! This workshop can provide some ideas to help you make meals easy and healthy.

Source: North Dakota State University Extension Service, *Good Nutrition for Busy Families.* http://www.ag.ndsu.edu/pubs/yf/foods/fn1432.pdf

Talking Points—Purpose of the Workshop (2–3 minutes)

- Today's workshop and handouts will give you tips for making meals and snacks that are both healthy and can be prepared quickly.

- This workshop is based on the *Dietary Guidelines for Americans, 2010* and the *2008 Physical Activity Guidelines for Americans.* The Dietary Guidelines provide science-based advice for making food choices that promote good health and a healthy weight and help prevent disease. The Physical Activity Guidelines provide recommendations on the amount, types, and level of intensity of physical activity needed to achieve and maintain good health.

- The Dietary Guidelines provide these selected consumer messages. More information about the messages can be found at http://www.ChooseMyPlate.gov.
  - *Balancing Calories*
    - ✓ Enjoy your food, but eat less.
    - ✓ Avoid oversized portions.
  - *Foods to Increase*
    - ✓ Make half your plate fruits and vegetables.
    - ✓ Make at least half your grains whole grains.
    - ✓ Switch to fat-free or low-fat (1%) milk.
  - *Foods to Decrease*
    - ✓ Compare sodium in foods like soup, bread, and frozen meals—and choose foods with lower numbers.
    - ✓ Drink water instead of sugary drinks.
  - Healthy eating and physical activity work hand in hand to help us live healthier lives. The Physical Activity Guidelines recommend that adults be physically active for at least 2 hours and 30 minutes each week—children need 60 minutes each day.
    - ✓ You can stay physically active by doing activities such as walking, dancing, bicycling, or gardening and by reducing the amount of time you spend sitting.

Talking Points—Learning Objectives (2–3 minutes)

1. Learn tips for preparing meals quickly and how to stock your pantry.

2. Learn how to make healthy selections when eating out.

3. Learn how to use a slow cooker to prepare easy, healthy meals.

Talking Points—Handout: Quick, Healthy Meals and Snacks (5 minutes)

Eating at Home Tips

- Stock your pantry or freezer with whole-wheat pasta or rice, cans of no-salt-added crushed tomatoes, spices, garlic, frozen chicken breasts, canned fish, and frozen vegetables.

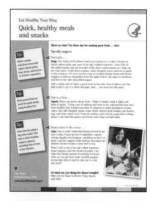

- Plan to use leftovers from one meal, such as cooked vegetables and meats, in a new and easy recipe for the next night, such as burritos or an omelet.

- Save time in the kitchen by using a slow cooker to make two or three healthy suppers at once.

Talking Points—Handout: My Shopping List (5 minutes)

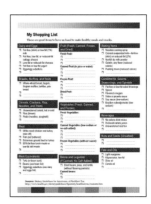

- It is easy to put together a quick meal if you have food already in your pantry. Look to buy nonperishable items on sale, such as low-sodium canned goods.

- Keep a note on the refrigerator to list items as you need them. You also may want to arrange your shopping list and coupons to fit the layout of the grocery store for a faster shopping trip.

Healthy, Quick Meal Ideas—*Remind participants to use MyPlate for balanced meals.*

- Serve pre-cut vegetables and low-fat ranch dressing, canned peaches in 100% juice or fresh fruit, and low-fat milk.

- Serve breakfast for dinner—omelet with vegetables (try mushrooms, red pepper, onions, spinach, tomatoes, etc.), fat-free or low-fat milk, and fruit.

- Serve low-sodium canned soup, a side salad with low-fat or fat-free dressing, and low-fat yogurt.

Healthy Snack Ideas—*You may choose to discuss these before or after the stretch break. If before the stretch break, challenge the group to come up with other ideas.*

- "Ants on a log" (celery with peanut butter and raisins)

- Fresh or canned fruit (in 100% juice, not syrup) with fat-free or low-fat vanilla yogurt

- Whole-grain crackers with fat-free or low-fat cheese

- Whole-wheat bread or apple slices with peanut butter

- Quesadillas (fat-free or low-fat cheese on a whole-wheat tortilla)

- Unsalted pretzels or air-popped popcorn

- Baked tortilla chips and salsa

- Whole-wheat pita bread or cut up vegetables (peppers, carrots, etc.) with hummus

- Fat-free or low-fat milk or water instead of sugary fruit drinks and soda

TIP: Put fresh fruit in a bowl at eye level in the refrigerator or on the kitchen counter. It will be easier to see and grab for a quick snack.

Video: Make It Fast, Make It Good (2–3 minutes)

Stretch Break (5 minutes)

"Name Your Favorite Healthy Snacks"

Ask participants to find a partner and walk around the room, with one partner sharing the name of his or her favorite healthy snack and how to prepare it. After 30 seconds, ask partners to switch roles, so that the other partners can share. After each partner has shared, ask them to find a new partner and repeat the exercise—this time sharing a different healthy snack idea. Be sure that participants keep moving/walking the entire time. Ask participants to share their creative ideas with the group.

Talking Points—Handouts: Tips for Eating Out and Tips for Choosing Healthier Foods at Restaurants (5–10 minutes)

Tips for Reducing Portions

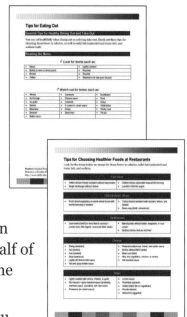

- Choose "child's size" portions if possible or choose the smallest size available.

- Eat half of your meal at the restaurant and save the other half for tomorrow's lunch.

- Order an appetizer-sized portion or a side dish instead of an entrée.

- Share a main dish with a friend.

- Resign from the "clean your plate club"—when you've eaten enough, leave the rest. Or, ask your server to package up half of your meal when it arrives so you won't be tempted to eat the entire portion.

- Order an item from the menu instead of heading for the "all-you-can-eat" buffet.

Tips for Reducing Calories

- For a beverage, ask for water or order fat-free or low-fat milk, unsweetened tea, or other drinks without added sugars.

- Load sandwiches/subs/pizza with veggies rather than cheese.

- Ask for whole-wheat bread for sandwiches, and ask that it not be buttered.

- In a restaurant, start your meal with a salad packed with veggies, to help control hunger and feel satisfied sooner.

- Ask for salad dressing to be served on the side. Then use only as much as you need.

Activity—Choose One Ahead of Time (5–10 minutes)

1. **Slow Cooking:** Demonstrate how to use a slow cooker and the amount of time it can save in preparing a healthy meal. Put chopped vegetables on the bottom of the slow cooker bowl, then place skinless chicken breasts or lean beef on top, add a can of no-salt-added diced tomatoes, oregano, and garlic. Turn the slow cooker on and let it cook during the workshop.

   Supplies necessary: slow cooker, chopped green, red, or yellow peppers, onion, zucchini, carrots, 1 pound of skinless chicken breasts or lean beef, 14½-oz can of no-salt-added diced tomatoes, 1½ teaspoons oregano, two cloves of minced garlic, can opener. See Note in Lesson Plan about suggested timing for completing this activity.

   Note: You will need to chop the vegetables ahead of time (before class). Also, if you will be presenting the workshop in a location without a sink to wash your hands after placing the meat in the slow cooker, you can put the chicken/beef into a sealed plastic bag and then empty the bag into the slow cooker without touching the meat. See Appendix for additional information on food safety and recipes.

2. **Tips for Eating Out:** Go over the *Tips for Eating Out* and *Tips for Choosing Healthier Foods at Restaurants* handouts, reviewing the tips for the types of restaurants located near where participants live. Then, distribute menus from local restaurants that serve some of these kinds of food. Assign participants to small groups, give each group a menu, and ask them to circle/highlight the healthiest selections.

   Supplies necessary: variety of ethnically diverse menus from local restaurants, highlighters or pens to highlight or circle healthy options

Talking Points—Handout: Slow Cooker Tips and Recipes (5–10 minutes)

Not sure what to make for dinner? In a rush when you get home at the end of the day? Try a slow cooker! A few minutes of prep in the morning is all you need for a simple meal for dinner. Try these recipes for "Refried" Beans and Turkey Chili made in a slow cooker.

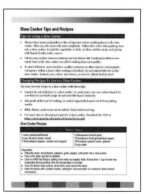

Why Use a Slow Cooker?

Using a slow cooker can be a quick, simple, and inexpensive way to prepare meals for your family, plus:

- Saves electricity! A slow cooker uses less electricity than an oven and doesn't overheat your kitchen.

- Saves money! You can use less-expensive cuts of meat because the slow cooker makes them tender.

- Saves time! Slow cookers usually allow one-step meal preparation and easy clean-up.

Talking Points—Increasing Physical Activity (1–2 minutes)

- The *Physical Activity Guidelines for Americans* recommend that everyone engage in regular physical activity for health benefits.

- Here are the recommendations for adults:

	Moderate Activity	Vigorous Activity
Types of Activity	Walking briskly, biking on flat ground, line dancing, gardening	Jumping rope, basketball, soccer, swimming laps, aerobic dance
Amount	If you choose activities at a **moderate** level, do at least **2 hours and 30 minutes a week**	If you choose activities at a **vigorous** level, do at least **1 hour and 15 minutes a week**

- You can combine moderate and vigorous activities. In general, 1 minute of vigorous activity is equal to 2 minutes of moderate activity.

- Children need **60 minutes of physical activity each day.**

- **TODAY'S TIP:** Increase physical activity by adding a new activity or spending more time doing an activity you already enjoy.

  ✓ Pick activities that you like to do and that fit into your life.

  ✓ Keep track of your physical activity and gradually increase it to meet the recommendations.

- Consider signing up for the Presidential Active Lifestyle Award (PALA+) to help you track your physical activity and take small steps to improve your eating habits.

- If you are active for 30 minutes a day, 5 days a week for 6 out of 8 weeks, and choose one healthy eating goal each week to work toward, you'll be awarded the PALA+ and receive Presidential recognition! (See http://www.presidentschallenge.org). See handout in Appendix for more information.

Talking Points—Handouts: MyPlate and 10 Tips (2 minutes)

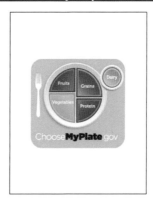
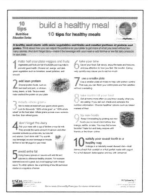

Talking Points—Wrap-Up/Q&A (5 minutes)

Things to Try at Home

- Next time you go to a restaurant, order a healthy dish using the tips for choosing items lower in calories, solid fats (saturated and trans fat), and sodium.
- Increase the total amount of time you spend doing physical activity.

Complete Evaluation Form (5 minutes)

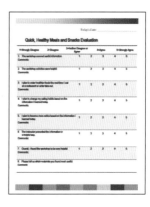

Workshop 2 ● Handouts

Eat Healthy Your Way
Quick, healthy meals and snacks

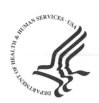

Short on time? Try these tips for making good foods . . . fast!

Speedy suppers

◀ **Pasta plus . . .**

Greg: One thing you'll always find in my pantry is a couple of boxes of whole-wheat pasta and cans of no-salt crushed tomatoes. I don't like all the added sugars and salt in some of the store's pasta sauces, so I make up my own sauce. I add dried oregano, basil, chopped onion, and lots of garlic to the tomatoes. I'll even toss in a bag of cooked chicken breast and frozen veggies or leftover vegetables from the night before. My sauce is nutritious and low in fat, salt, and added sugars.

Add a salad, and we have a good meal in less time than it takes to get the kids ready to go to a drive-through. And . . . my sons love this meal.

◀ **Fish in a flash . . .**

Aponi: Here's my motto about food—"Make it simple, make it right, and make it quick." I keep cans of salmon and tuna in my cupboard because they have healthy fats. It takes less than 15 minutes to make up salmon or tuna cakes. Just add chopped onion, some whole-wheat bread crumbs, one beaten egg, and some celery seed. Form the patties, and cook in a pan with cooking spray. Cook until the patties are brown and crispy on both sides.

◀ **Slow cooker to the rescue . . .**

Anh: Once a week I make big batches of food in my slow cooker. I chop up lots of vegetables—carrots, onions, squash, sweet peppers—anything we have on hand. I put the veggies on the bottom, then place my skinless chicken breasts or lean beef on top.

Then, I add a can of no-salt-added tomatoes, some oregano, and two cloves of garlic. I do other fun things instead of cooking for hours. And, we can get three tasty, healthy suppers in less time than it used to take me to cook one meal!

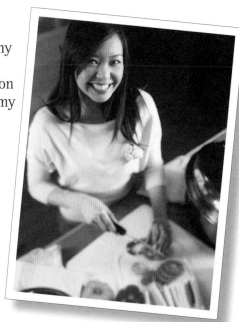

So what are you doing for dinner tonight?
Why not try what works for Greg, Aponi, and Anh?

Tip:

Make a quick, nutritious meal with whole-wheat pasta, lean meats, and frozen or leftover vegetables.

Tip:

Keep canned fish on hand for quick meals using healthy fats.

Tip:

Save time by using a big slow cooker. Get two or three healthy suppers without spending lots of time in the kitchen.

▼ For more information, visit
www.healthfinder.gov

(turn over please)

Small changes can make a large difference

Hearty, healthy lunches in a snap

- **Sandwich lover?** Choose lean protein fillings, such as grilled chicken or tuna. Make nonmeat sandwiches with peanut butter, low-fat cheese, sliced hard-boiled eggs, or fat-free refried beans.
- **Load your sandwich with veggies.** Along with the standard greens and tomatoes . . . try sliced cucumbers, green peppers, or zucchini strips for added crunch.
- **Pick whole grains!** Try whole-grain or 100% whole-wheat breads, tortilla wraps, English muffins, and pita pockets instead of white breads or buns.
- **Green salads, anyone?** Add lean meats along with fruits, beans, and nuts to your green salads. Try dried cranberries, cut-up fruit, kidney beans, walnuts, and almonds.

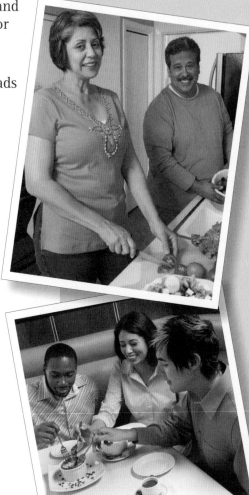

On the run? Healthier fast food or drive-through choices

Skip the meal deals and size upgrades

Calories can really add up when you get the larger size sandwiches, fried foods, and soft drinks.

Check off what you will try to cut the calories when eating out:

- Get the regular or child-sized hamburger and load it with lettuce, tomato, and onions.
- Cut a larger burger or sandwich in half. Eat half now, and refrigerate half for tomorrow's lunch.
- Get the small size turkey or grilled chicken sub instead of the large one. Load it with veggies—spinach, tomatoes, cucumbers, and onions.
- Drink water, or low-fat or fat-free milk, instead of whole milk, fruit drinks, or a soft drink.

Go healthier

- Order a side salad with low-fat or fat-free dressing instead of fries. Or share an order of small fries with a friend.
- Use mustard, or low-fat or fat-free mayo, instead of regular mayo.
- Choose the green beans or raw carrots instead of coleslaw. Order a small baked potato with salsa instead of mashed potatoes and gravy.
- Order a thin-crust vegetable pizza with a side salad instead of a deep-dish meat or double cheese pizza.
- Save foods like cakes, pies, and brownies as an occasional treat. Order fruit instead. Or share one dessert.

My Shopping List

These are good items to have on hand to make healthy meals and snacks.

Dairy and Eggs

- ☐ Fat-free (skim) or low-fat (1%) milk
- ☐ Fat-free, low-fat, or reduced-fat cottage cheese
- ☐ Low-fat or reduced-fat cheeses
- ☐ Fat-free or low-fat yogurt
- ☐ Eggs/egg substitute
- ☐ _____

Breads, Muffins, and Rolls

- ☐ Whole-wheat bread, bagels, English muffins, tortillas, pita bread
- ☐ _____
- ☐ _____

Cereals, Crackers, Rice, Noodles, and Pasta

- ☐ Unsweetened cereal, hot or cold
- ☐ Rice (brown)
- ☐ Pasta (noodles, spaghetti)
- ☐ _____

Meat

- ☐ White meat chicken and turkey (skin off)
- ☐ Fish (not battered)
- ☐ Extra-lean ground beef or turkey
- ☐ 95% fat-free lunch meats or low-fat deli meats
- ☐ _____

Meat Equivalents

- ☐ Tofu (or bean curd)
- ☐ Beans (see bean list)
- ☐ Eggs/egg substitute (see dairy and eggs list)
- ☐ _____

Fruit (Fresh, Canned, Frozen, and Dried)

Fresh Fruit:
- ☐ _____
- ☐ _____
- ☐ _____

Canned Fruit (in juice or water):
- ☐ _____
- ☐ _____
- ☐ _____

Frozen Fruit:
- ☐ _____
- ☐ _____
- ☐ _____

Dried Fruit:
- ☐ _____
- ☐ _____

Vegetables (Fresh, Canned, and Frozen)

Fresh Vegetables:
- ☐ _____
- ☐ _____
- ☐ _____

Canned Vegetables (low-sodium or no-salt-added):
- ☐ _____
- ☐ _____
- ☐ _____

Frozen Vegetables (without sauce):
- ☐ _____
- ☐ _____
- ☐ _____

Beans and Legumes (If Canned, No Salt Added)

- ☐ Dried beans, peas, and lentils (without flavoring packets)

Canned beans:
- ☐ _____
- ☐ _____

Baking Items

- ☐ Nonstick cooking spray
- ☐ Canned evaporated milk—fat-free (skim) or reduced-fat (2%)
- ☐ Nonfat dry milk powder
- ☐ Gelatin, any flavor (reduced calorie)
- ☐ Pudding mixes (reduced calorie)
- ☐ _____

Condiments, Sauces, Seasonings, and Spreads

- ☐ Fat-free or low-fat salad dressings
- ☐ Spices
- ☐ Flavored vinegars
- ☐ Salsa or picante sauce
- ☐ Soy sauce (low-sodium)
- ☐ Bouillon cubes/granules (low-sodium)
- ☐ _____

Beverages

- ☐ No-calorie drink mixes
- ☐ Reduced-calorie juices
- ☐ Unsweetened iced tea
- ☐ _____

Nuts and Seeds (Unsalted)

- ☐ _____
- ☐ _____

Fats and Oils

- ☐ Light margarine
- ☐ Mayonnaise, low-fat
- ☐ Olive oil
- ☐ Canola oil
- ☐ _____

Source: Dietary Guidelines for Americans, *A Healthier You.*
http://www.health.gov/dietaryguidelines/dga2005/healthieryou/contents.htm

Tips for Eating Out

General Tips for Healthy Dining Out and Take-Out

You can eat healthfully when dining out or ordering take-out. Check out these tips for choosing items lower in calories, as well as-solid fats (saturated and *trans* fat), and sodium (salt).

Reading the Menu

👍 Look for terms such as:

• Baked	• Lightly sautéed
• Boiled (in wine or lemon juice)	• Poached
• Broiled	• Roasted
• Grilled	• Steamed in its own juice (au jus)

👎 Watch out for terms such as:

• Alfredo	• Casserole	• Escalloped
• Au fromage	• Cheese sauce	• Fried
• Au gratin	• Creamed	• Gravy
• Basted	• In cream or cream sauce	• Hollandaise
• Béarnaise	• Crispy	• Pastry crust
• Breaded	• Deep fried	• Pot pie
• Butter sauce		

Source: Adapted from National Heart, Lung, and Blood Institute (NHLBI), *Aim for a Healthy Weight: Maintaining a Healthy Weight On the Go—A Pocket Guide,* page 12.
http://www.nhlbi.nih.gov/health/public/heart/obesity/AIM_Pocket_Guide_tagged.pdf

Tips for Choosing Healthier Foods at Restaurants

Look for the terms below on menus for items lower in calories, solid fats (saturated and *trans* fat), and sodium.

Fast Food

- Grilled chicken breast sandwich without mayonnaise
- Single hamburger without cheese
- Grilled chicken salad with reduced-fat dressing
- Low-fat or fat-free yogurt

Deli/Sandwich Shops

- Fresh sliced vegetables on whole-wheat bread with low-fat dressing or mustard
- Turkey breast sandwich with mustard, lettuce, and tomato
- Bean soup (lentil, minestrone)

Steakhouses

- Lean broiled beef (no more than 6 ounces)— London broil, filet mignon, round and flank steaks
- Baked potato without butter, margarine, or sour cream
- Seafood dishes that are not fried

Chinese

- Zheng (steamed)
- Gun (boiled)
- Kao (roasted)
- Shao (barbecue)
- Lightly stir-fried in mild sauce
- Hot and spicy tomato sauce
- Reduced-sodium soy, hoisin, and oyster sauce
- Dishes without MSG added
- Bean curd (tofu)
- Moo shu vegetables, chicken, or shrimp
- Hot mustard sauce

Italian

- Lightly sautéed with onions, shallots, or garlic
- Red sauces—spicy marinara sauce (arrabiata), marinara sauce, cacciatore, red clam sauce
- Primavera (no cream sauce)
- Lemon sauce
- Florentine (spinach)
- Grilled (often fish or vegetables)
- Piccata (lemon)
- Manzanne (eggplant)

Middle Eastern	
• Fava beans or chickpeas • Basted with tomato sauce	• Couscous (grain) • Rice or bulgur (cracked wheat)

Japanese	
• House salad with fresh ginger and cellophane (clear rice) noodles • Chicken, fish, or shrimp teriyaki, broiled in sauce	• Soba noodles, often used in soups • Yakimono (broiled) • Tofu (or bean curd) • Nabemono (soup/stew)

Indian	
• Tikka (pan roasted) • Cooked with or marinated in yogurt • Saag (with spinach) • Masala (mixture of spices)	• Tandoori (chicken marinated in yogurt with spices) • Pullao (Basmati rice)

Thai	
• Fish sauce	• Hot sauce

Source: Adapted from National Heart, Lung, and Blood Institute (NHLBI), *Aim for a Healthy Weight: Maintaining a Healthy Weight On the Go—A Pocket Guide,* pages 14–18.
http://www.nhlbi.nih.gov/health/public/heart/obesity/AIM_Pocket_Guide_tagged.pdf

Slow Cooker Tips and Recipes

Tips for Using a Slow Cooker

- Always thaw meat and poultry in the refrigerator before cooking them in the slow cooker. This way, the meat will cook completely. Follow this order when putting food into a slow cooker: (1) put the vegetables in first, (2) then add the meat, and (3) top with liquid (broth, water, sauce).

- Fill the slow cooker between halfway and two-thirds full. Cooking too little or too much food in the slow cooker can affect cooking time and quality.

- To store leftovers, move food to a smaller container to allow food to cool properly; refrigerate within 2 hours after cooking is finished. Do not reheat leftovers in the slow cooker. Instead, use a stove, microwave, or oven to reheat food to 165°F.

Changing Recipes To Use in a Slow Cooker

Try your favorite recipe in a slow cooker with these tips:

- Liquids do not boil away in a slow cooker. In most cases, you can reduce liquids by one-third to one-half (soups do not need the liquid reduced).

- Add pasta at the end of cooking, or cook it separately to prevent it from getting mushy.

- Milk, cheese, and cream can be added 1 hour before serving.

- For more tips on changing recipes for a slow cooker, download the PDF at http://www.ag.ndsu.edu/pubs/yf/foods/fn1511.pdf.

Slow Cooker Recipes

"Refried" Beans	
1 onion, peeled and halved 3 cups dry pinto beans, rinsed ½ fresh jalapeno pepper, seeded and chopped	2 tablespoons minced garlic 1¾ teaspoons fresh ground black pepper 1/8 teaspoon ground cumin, optional 9 cups water
Preparation: • Place the onion, rinsed beans, jalapeno, garlic, pepper, and cumin into a slow cooker. • Pour in the water and stir to combine. • Cook on HIGH for 8 hours, adding more water as needed. Note: if more than 1 cup of water has evaporated during cooking, then the temperature is too high. • Once the beans have cooked, strain them, and reserve the liquid. • Mash the beans with a potato masher, adding the reserved water as needed to attain desired consistency.	

Quick Tip—"Refried" Beans

- Try these beans in tacos and burritos. Or, use as a dip for your favorite veggies!
- You also could use it as a spread on your favorite sandwich.

Turkey Chili	
1¼ pounds lean ground turkey 1 large onion, chopped 1 garlic clove, minced 1½ cups frozen corn kernels 1 red bell pepper, chopped 1 green bell pepper, chopped 1 (28-oz.) can crushed tomatoes	1 (15-oz.) can black beans, rinsed and drained 1 (8-oz.) can tomato sauce 1 (1.25-oz.) package chili seasoning mix ½ teaspoon salt Toppings: fat-free or reduced fat shredded cheese, finely chopped red onion

Preparation:
- Cook first three ingredients in a large skillet over medium-high heat, stirring until turkey crumbles and is no longer pink; drain.
- Spoon mixture into a slow cooker; stir in corn and next seven ingredients until well blended.
- Cook at HIGH 4 to 5 hours or at LOW 6 to 8 hours.
- Serve with desired toppings.

Quick Tip—Turkey Chili

Make extra chili for another meal. Use the rest to:

- Top baked potatoes.

- Make an easy casserole by combining cooked whole wheat pasta shells with chili.

- Make a quick and easy taco salad by topping lettuce with chili, diced tomatoes and shredded chees

Source: Tips adapted from USDA's Slow Cookers and Food Safety
http://www.fsis.usda.gov/Fact_Sheets/Focus_On_Slow_Cooker_Safety/index.asp
Recipes: http://allrecipes.com/recipe/refried-beans-without-the-refry/detail.aspx and
http://www.myrecipes.com/recipe/slow-cooker-turkey-chili-10000001176221/

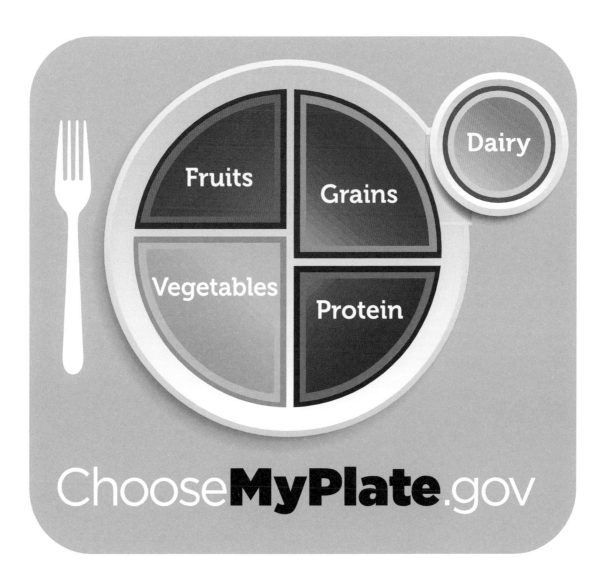

ChooseMyPlate.gov

10 tips

Nutrition Education Series

build a healthy meal

10 **tips** for healthy meals

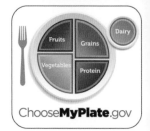
ChooseMyPlate.gov

A healthy meal starts with more vegetables and fruits and smaller portions of protein and grains. Think about how you can adjust the portions on your plate to get more of what you need without too many calories. And don't forget dairy—make it the beverage with your meal or add fat-free or low-fat dairy products to your plate.

1 make half your plate veggies and fruits
Vegetables and fruits are full of nutrients and may help to promote good health. Choose red, orange, and dark-green vegetables such as tomatoes, sweet potatoes, and broccoli.

2 add lean protein
Choose protein foods, such as lean beef and pork, or chicken, turkey, beans, or tofu. Twice a week, make seafood the protein on your plate.

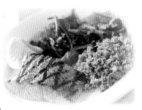

3 include whole grains
Aim to make at least half your grains whole grains. Look for the words "100% whole grain" or "100% whole wheat" on the food label. Whole grains provide more nutrients, like fiber, than refined grains.

4 don't forget the dairy
Pair your meal with a cup of fat-free or low-fat milk. They provide the same amount of calcium and other essential nutrients as whole milk, but less fat and calories. Don't drink milk? Try soymilk (soy beverage) as your beverage or include fat-free or low-fat yogurt in your meal.

5 avoid extra fat
Using heavy gravies or sauces will add fat and calories to otherwise healthy choices. For example, steamed broccoli is great, but avoid topping it with cheese sauce. Try other options, like a sprinkling of low-fat parmesan cheese or a squeeze of lemon.

6 take your time
Savor your food. Eat slowly, enjoy the taste and textures, and pay attention to how you feel. Be mindful. Eating very quickly may cause you to eat too much.

7 use a smaller plate
Use a smaller plate at meals to help with portion control. That way you can finish your entire plate and feel satisfied without overeating.

8 take control of your food
Eat at home more often so you know exactly what you are eating. If you eat out, check and compare the nutrition information. Choose healthier options such as baked instead of fried.

9 try new foods
Keep it interesting by picking out new foods you've never tried before, like mango, lentils, or kale. You may find a new favorite! Trade fun and tasty recipes with friends or find them online.

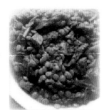

10 satisfy your sweet tooth in a healthy way
Indulge in a naturally sweet dessert dish—fruit! Serve a fresh fruit cocktail or a fruit parfait made with yogurt. For a hot dessert, bake apples and top with cinnamon.

USDA
United States Department of Agriculture
Center for Nutrition Policy and Promotion

DG TipSheet No. 7
June 2011
USDA is an equal opportunity provider and employer.

Go to www.ChooseMyPlate.gov for more information.

Quick, Healthy Meals and Snacks Evaluation

1=Strongly Disagree	2=Disagree	3=Neither Disagree or Agree		4=Agree		5=Strongly Agree
1. The workshop covered useful information. Comments:		1	2	3	4	5
2. The workshop activities were helpful. Comments:		1	2	3	4	5
3. I plan to order healthier foods the next time I eat at a restaurant or order take-out. Comments:		1	2	3	4	5
4. I plan to change my eating habits based on the information I learned today. Comments:		1	2	3	4	5
5. I plan to become more active based on the information I learned today. Comments:		1	2	3	4	5
6. The instructor presented the information in a helpful way. Comments:		1	2	3	4	5
7. Overall, I found the workshop to be very helpful. Comments:		1	2	3	4	5

8. Please tell us which materials you found most useful.
Comments:

Workshop 3

Eating Healthy on a Budget

Eat Healthy ● *Be Active*
Community Workshops

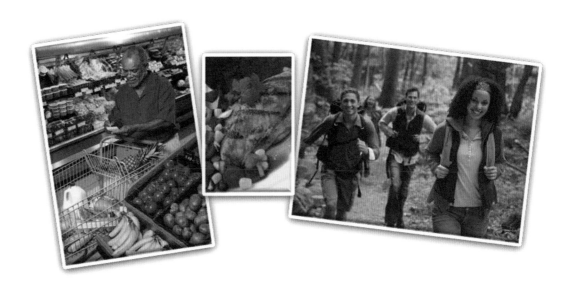

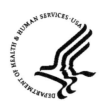

OFFICE OF
DISEASE
PREVENTION AND
HEALTH
PROMOTION

Instructor Guide

Before Workshop Begins

- Thoroughly read entire workshop and become familiar with the lesson plan.
- Gather materials needed for the icebreaker and activity.
  - *Icebreaker:* Store-brand canned fruit in unsweetened fruit juice, name-brand canned fruit in unsweetened fruit juice, can opener, disposable bowls and spoons
  - *Activity:* Sales circulars from several local grocery stores, pens, copies of *Grocery List* handout
- Photocopy handouts (one per participant):
  1. Eating Healthy on a Budget (2 pages)
  2. Weekly Meal Planner (2 pages)
  3. Grocery List (1 page)
  4. MyPlate/10 Tips to Eat Better on a Budget (2 pages)
  5. Workshop Evaluation (1 page)

Workshop Outline

The workshop should last ~1 hour, including activities.

- Icebreaker activity (5 minutes)—do this while people are coming into the workshop
- Introduction (5 minutes)
  - Explain the purpose of the workshop
  - Review the Learning Objectives
- **Objective 1:** Learn the three steps for healthy eating on a budget—planning, purchasing, and preparing (10–15 minutes)
  - Review handout: *Healthy Eating on a Budget*
- Video: *Budget Stretching Healthy Meals* (2–3 minutes)
- Stretch Break (5 minutes)

- **Objective 2:** Learn how to plan meals and snacks ahead of time (10–15 minutes)
  - Review handout: *Weekly Meal Planner*
- Activity (5–10 minutes)
  - Review handout: *Grocery List*
- Increasing Physical Activity (1–2 minutes)
- Review handout *MyPlate* and how to use *10 Tips to Eat Better on a Budget* (2 minutes)
- Wrap-up/Q&A (5 minutes)
  - Reminders of things to try at home:
    - Plan meals for the week using sale items from the store circular
    - Choose moderate- or vigorous-intensity physical activity
- Ask participants to complete the evaluation form (5 minutes)

Additional Activity—*Note:* This would need to be planned ahead of time and scheduled for a time after the workshop:

Grocery Store Field Trip: Your local supermarket may be able to arrange a store tour for your group with its registered dietitian (RD). More information about this service may be available on the store's Web site or by contacting the store manager or RD. Also, the community outreach department of your local hospital may be able to arrange for an RD to provide this service. While at the store, have participants use their shopping lists; you can help them locate the healthy sale items and search the aisles for other healthy foods.

Workshop Lesson Plan

Icebreaker Activity—Taste Testing (5 minutes)

Generic vs. Brand Taste Test: Compare store-brand canned fruit in unsweetened fruit juice with name-brand canned fruit in unsweetened fruit juice.

Supplies necessary: Store-brand canned fruit in unsweetened fruit juice, name-brand canned fruit in unsweetened fruit juice, can opener, disposable bowls and spoons

Talking Points—Purpose of the Workshop (2–3 minutes)

- Today's workshop and handouts will give you tips for making meals and snacks that are both healthy and allow you to stay within your budget.

- This workshop is based on the *Dietary Guidelines for Americans, 2010* and the *2008 Physical Activity Guidelines for Americans*. The Dietary Guidelines provide science-based advice for making food choices that promote good health and a healthy weight and help prevent disease. The Physical Activity Guidelines provide recommendations on the amount, types, and level of intensity of physical activity needed to achieve and maintain good health.

- The Dietary Guidelines provide these selected consumer messages. More information about the messages can be found at http://www.ChooseMyPlate.gov.

  - *Balancing Calories*

    ✓ Enjoy your food, but eat less.

    ✓ Avoid oversized portions.

  - *Foods to Increase*

    ✓ Make half your plate fruits and vegetables.

    ✓ Make at least half your grains whole grains.

    ✓ Switch to fat-free or low-fat (1%) milk.

  - *Foods to Decrease*

    ✓ Compare sodium in foods like soup, bread, and frozen meals—and choose foods with lower numbers.

    ✓ Drink water instead of sugary drinks.

  - Healthy eating and physical activity work hand in hand to help us live healthier lives. The Physical Activity Guidelines recommend that adults be physically active for at least 2 hours and 30 minutes each week—children need 60 minutes each day.

    ✓ You can stay physically active by doing activities such as walking, dancing, bicycling, or gardening and by reducing the amount of time you spend sitting.

Talking Points—Learning Objectives (2–3 minutes)

1. Learn the three steps for healthy eating on a budget—planning, purchasing, and preparing.

2. Learn how to plan meals and snacks ahead of time.

Talking Points—Handout: Eating Healthy on a Budget (10–15 minutes)

Step 1. Plan ahead before you shop.

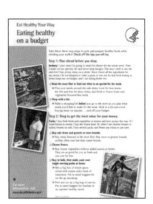

- Plan meals and snacks for the week according to a budget.

- Find quick and easy recipes online.

- Include meals that will "stretch" expensive food items (stews, casseroles, stir-fries).

- Make a grocery list.

- Check for sales and coupons in the local paper or online and consider discount stores.

- Ask about a loyalty card at your grocery store.

Step 2. Shop to get the most value out of your budget.

- Buy groceries when you are not hungry and when you are not too rushed.

- Remember to purchase refrigerated and freezer food items last and store them promptly when you get home. Proper refrigeration will help food last longer.

- Stick to the grocery list, and stay out of the aisles that don't contain things on your list.

- Cut coupons from newspaper circulars or online and bring them to the store with you. Try to combine coupons with items on sale for more savings!

- Find and compare unit prices listed on shelves to get the best price.

- Buy store brands if cheaper.

- Purchase some items in bulk or as family packs, which usually cost less.

- Choose fresh fruits and vegetables in season; buy canned vegetables with less salt.

- Precut fruits and vegetables, individual cups of yogurt, and instant rice and hot cereal are convenient, but usually cost more.

- Good low-cost items year-round include:

  – Protein—beans (garbanzo, black, kidney, northern, lima)

  – Vegetables—carrots, greens, potatoes

  – Fruit—apples, bananas, 100% frozen orange juice

  – Grains—brown rice, oats

  – Dairy—fat-free or low-fat (1%) milk

Step 3. Make cost-cutting meals.

- Some meal items can be prepared in advance; precook on days when you have time.

- Double or triple up on recipes and freeze meal-sized containers of soups and casseroles or divide into individual portions and freeze.

- Try a few meatless meals by featuring beans and peas, or try "no-cook" meals like salads.

- Incorporate leftovers into a meal later in the week.

Video: Budget Stretching Healthy Meals (2–3 minutes)

Stretch Break (5 minutes)

"Beans" (celebrating beans because they are inexpensive and packed with nutrients)

Have participants stand up and spread out to allow space for them to move. The facilitator calls out names of beans, and the participants do set actions to each.

- Baked beans—make a small shape with your body
- Broad beans—make a wide, stretched-out shape
- String beans—make a tall, string-like shape
- Jumping beans—jump up and down (say "small jumping beans" for small jumps and "big jumping beans" for the opposite)
- Chili beans—shiver and shake as if it were cold
- French beans—do the *can-can*, with high kicks

Talking Points—Stretch Break

- Dry beans will be less expensive than canned beans. Remember to rinse canned beans to reduce the sodium.

- Kidney, lima, garbanzo, and northern beans are the least expensive beans.

Talking Points—Handout: Weekly Meal Planner (5–10 minutes)

Tips for Making Changes

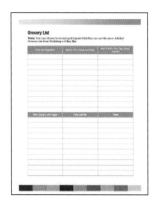

- Cook large portions ahead of time, or use your leftovers to create a second meal.

    – Most leftovers can be used to make tasty burritos (put everything in a whole-wheat tortilla with a little low-fat cheese).

    – Add your leftover meat and vegetables to a large green salad.

- Go meatless a few meals a week.

- Drink water instead of high-calorie and costly beverages.

- Decrease the amount of less healthy foods (soda, cookies, chips, etc.) you buy, and see how much you will save while becoming healthier!

Activity—Handout: Grocery List (5–10 minutes)

1. **Healthy Shopping List:** Pass out sales circulars for neighborhood grocery stores, and ask participants to fill in foods on their *Grocery List* handouts based on healthy items on sale.

2. **Supplies necessary:** Sales circulars from several local grocery stores, pens, copies of *Grocery List* handout.

Talking Points—Increasing Physical Activity (1–2 minutes)

- The *Physical Activity Guidelines for Americans* recommend that everyone engage in regular physical activity for health benefits.

- Here are the recommendations for adults:

	Moderate Activity	Vigorous Activity
Types of Activity	Walking briskly, biking on flat ground, line dancing, gardening	Jumping rope, basketball, soccer, swimming laps, aerobic dance
Amount	If you choose activities at a **moderate** level, do at least **2 hours and 30 minutes a week**	If you choose activities at a **vigorous** level, do at least **1 hour and 15 minutes a week**

- You can combine moderate and vigorous activities. In general, 1 minute of vigorous activity is equal to 2 minutes of moderate activity.

- Children need **60 minutes of physical activity each day.**

- **TODAY'S TIP:** Choose moderate-or vigorous-intensity physical activities.

  - ✓ **Moderate-intensity activities** include walking briskly, biking, dancing, general gardening, water aerobics, and canoeing.

  - ✓ **Vigorous-intensity activities** include aerobic dance, jumping rope, race walking, jogging, running, soccer, swimming fast or swimming laps, and riding a bike on hills or riding fast.

    - You can replace some or all of your moderate-intensity activity with vigorous activity.

    - With vigorous activities, you get similar health benefits in half the time it takes you with moderate ones.

  - ✓ Adults should include muscle-strengthening activities at least 2 days a week.

  - ✓ **Muscle-strengthening activities** include lifting weights, pushups, and sit-ups.

    - Choose activities that work all the different parts of the body—the legs, hips, back, chest, stomach, shoulders, and arms.

  - ✓ Encourage children to do muscle-strengthening activities, such as climbing, at least 3 days a week and bone-strengthening activities, such as jumping, at least 3 days a week.

- Consider signing up for the Presidential Active Lifestyle Award (PALA+) to help you track your physical activity and take small steps to improve your eating habits.

- If you are active for 30 minutes a day, 5 days a week for 6 out of 8 weeks, and choose one healthy eating goal each week to work toward, you'll be awarded the PALA+ and receive Presidential recognition! (See http://www.presidentschallenge.org) See handout in Appendix for more information.

Talking Points—Handouts: MyPlate and 10 Tips (2 minutes)

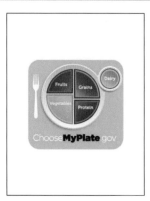
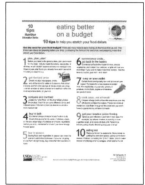

Talking Points—Wrap-up/Q&A (5 minutes)

Things to Try at Home

- Plan meals for the week using sale items from the store circular.
- Choose moderate- or vigorous-intensity physical activities.

Complete Evaluation Form (5 minutes)

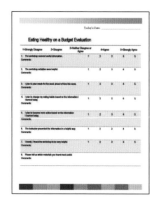

Workshop 3 ● Handouts

Eat Healthy Your Way
Eating healthy on a budget

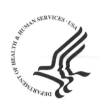

Take these three easy steps to pick and prepare healthy foods while minding your wallet! Check off the tips you will try.

Step 1: Plan ahead before you shop

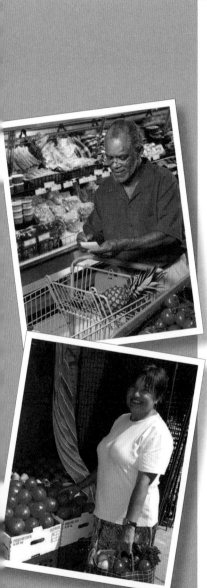

Rodney: I plan what I'm going to make for dinner for the whole week. Then I make out my grocery list and never shop hungry. This way I stick to my list and don't buy pricey items on a whim. Since I have all the ingredients for my meals, I'm not tempted to order a pizza or run out for fast food. Eating at home keeps me on budget, and I am eating better too.

❏ **Read the store flier to find out what is on special for the week.**

➤ Plan your meals around the sale items. Look for lean meats, fat-free and low-fat dairy items, and fresh or frozen fruits and vegetables featured that week.

❏ **Shop with a list.**

➤ Make a shopping list **before** you go to the store as you plan what meals you'd like to make for the week. Stick to a list and avoid buying items on impulse . . . and off your budget.

Step 2: Shop to get the most value for your money

Carla: I buy fresh fruits and vegetables in season and save money this way. If I want berries in winter, I buy the frozen kind. Or, when I see chicken breasts or turkey breasts on sale, I buy several packs and freeze any extras to use later.

❏ **Buy sale items and generic or store brands.**

➤ Buy items featured in the store flier. Buy store or generic brands, as they often cost less than name brands.

❏ **Choose frozen.**

➤ Buy frozen vegetables without added sauces or butter. They are as good for you as fresh and can cost far less.

❏ **Buy in bulk, then make your own single-serving packs at home.**

➤ Mix a big box of whole-grain cereal with raisins and a dash of cinnamon. Put in small baggies for on-the-go snacking.

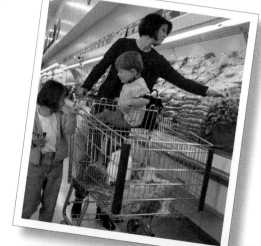

➤ Peel and cut up a big bag of carrots. Put in small baggies for lunches or an anytime healthy snack.

For more information, visit www.healthfinder.gov

(turn over please)

Small changes can make a large difference

Step 3: Make cost-cutting meals

Padma: Stretch your food dollars by making a second meal from leftovers—just add items you already have in your pantry. I took last night's leftover baked chicken and cut it into small pieces. Then I added a can of black beans, a chopped onion, two cloves of garlic, spices, and some chopped tomatoes. I made a low-cost, tasty meal in 15 minutes! And my family got a healthy dinner.

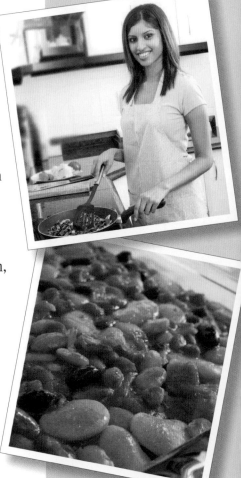

❑ **Make a second meal or a side dish from leftovers.**

Stretch your dollars by adding items you already have on hand to make a second meal or tasty side dish.

➤ Use leftover chicken or turkey in casseroles, soups, chili, stir-fries, or tacos.

➤ Use leftover brown rice in soups and casseroles. For a great side dish, cook brown rice with vegetables and a beaten egg in a pan coated with cooking spray.

➤ Add leftover cooked or raw vegetables to salads, omelets, or casseroles. Add the leftover veggies to whole-wheat pasta and water-packed tuna for a healthy, low-cost meal.

➤ Mix leftover fresh or canned fruit (packed in fruit juice) with low-fat plain yogurt or low-fat cottage cheese. Or put the fruit in oatmeal for a "good-for-you" breakfast.

❑ **Go meatless one or more days a week.**

➤ Replace meat with beans for a less costly way to get lean protein. Beans and brown rice are a nutritious way to stretch a dollar. Add lentils to soups. They are delicious, cook up quickly, and are packed with protein and fiber.

➤ Make breakfast for dinner! Prepare a vegetable omelet with eggs, spinach, tomatoes, mushrooms, and reduced-fat cheese. Serve with fruit and whole-wheat toast. Your kids will love the "upside-down day" that is budget-friendly for you!

❑ **Visit the Internet for recipe ideas.**

➤ Look on the Internet for many healthy recipes. Just type the words "healthy meals on a budget" in the search engine. Or visit **http://recipefinder.nal.usda.gov** to get recipe ideas that are easy on the wallet and good for your body.

> We hope these budget-stretching ideas will help you as you take steps to eat healthy.

ODPHP Publication No. U0050

Weekly Meal Planner

Use this tool to help plan healthier meals for your family. Below are ideas for healthier breakfasts, lunches, and dinners. Use the chart to plan meals for a week. Try to plan one dinner that uses leftovers from the night before and one that is meatless. Once you have the meals planned, write out your grocery list.

Ideas for Healthy Breakfasts

- 1 cup whole-grain cold or ½ cup whole-grain hot cereal, ½ cup fat-free or low-fat milk, and ½ cup fresh or frozen fruit, such as blueberries, sliced strawberries, or bananas.

- 2 slices whole-grain toast with 2 tablespoons peanut butter, 1 cup low-fat or fat-free yogurt, and ½ cup 100% juice.

- 2 scrambled eggs, 1 slice whole-grain toast, 1 cup fat-free or low-fat milk, and ½ cup sliced strawberries.

Ideas for Healthy Lunches

- 1 cup garden salad with 1 tablespoon fat-free or low-fat dressing and ½ turkey sandwich on whole-wheat bread with lettuce, tomato, and mustard.

- 1 cup broth or tomato-based soup and ½ lean roast beef sandwich on whole-wheat bread with lettuce, tomato, and mustard.

- 1 slice cheese or vegetable pizza made with low-fat cheese and small garden salad with 1 tablespoon fat-free or low-fat dressing.

Ideas for Healthy Dinners

- 3 ounces grilled honey mustard chicken, 1 cup green beans, and ½ cup wild rice.

- 3 ounces baked fish with lemon dill dressing, 1 cup herbed pasta, and 1 cup steamed frozen vegetables (such as mixed vegetables).

- 1 cup whole-wheat pasta with ½ cup tomato sauce, ½ cup steamed broccoli, 1 slice whole-grain bread, and ½ cup pineapple slices.

Day	Breakfast	Lunch	Dinner
Sunday			
Monday			
Tuesday			
Wednesday			
Thursday			
Friday			
Saturday			

Grocery List

Note: You may choose to remind participants that they can use the more detailed Grocery List from Workshop 2 if they like.

Fruits and Vegetables	Breads, Rice, Cereal, and Pasta	Meat, Poultry, Fish, Eggs, Beans, and Nuts

Milk, Cheese, and Yogurt	Fats and Oils	Other

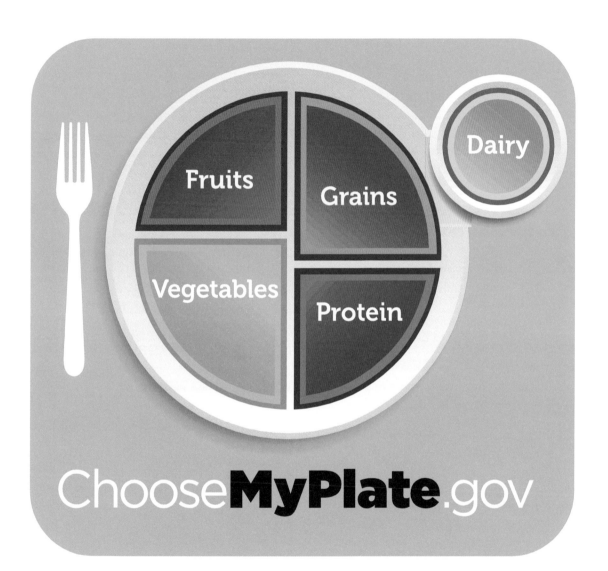

ChooseMyPlate.gov

10 tips
Nutrition Education Series

eating better on a budget

10 tips to help you stretch your food dollars

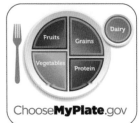

ChooseMyPlate.gov

Get the most for your food budget! There are many ways to save money on the foods that you eat. The three main steps are planning before you shop, purchasing the items at the best price, and preparing meals that stretch your food dollars.

1 plan, plan, plan!
Before you head to the grocery store, plan your meals for the week. Include meals like stews, casseroles, or stir-fries, which "stretch" expensive items into more portions. Check to see what foods you already have and make a list for what you need to buy.

2 get the best price
Check the local newspaper, online, and at the store for sales and coupons. Ask about a loyalty card for extra savings at stores where you shop. Look for specials or sales on meat and seafood—often the most expensive items on your list.

3 compare and contrast
Locate the "Unit Price" on the shelf directly below the product. Use it to compare different brands and different sizes of the same brand to determine which is more economical.

4 buy in bulk
It is almost always cheaper to buy foods in bulk. Smart choices are family packs of chicken, steak, or fish and larger bags of potatoes and frozen vegetables. Before you shop, remember to check if you have enough freezer space.

5 buy in season
Buying fruits and vegetables in season can lower the cost and add to the freshness! If you are not going to use them all right away, buy some that still need time to ripen.

6 convenience costs... go back to the basics
Convenience foods like frozen dinners, pre-cut vegetables, and instant rice, oatmeal, or grits will cost you more than if you were to make them from scratch. Take the time to prepare your own—and save!

7 easy on your wallet
Certain foods are typically low-cost options all year round. Try beans for a less expensive protein food. For vegetables, buy carrots, greens, or potatoes. As for fruits, apples and bananas are good choices.

8 cook once...eat all week!
Prepare a large batch of favorite recipes on your day off (double or triple the recipe). Freeze in individual containers. Use them throughout the week and you won't have to spend money on take-out meals.

9 get your creative juices flowing
Spice up your leftovers—use them in new ways. For example, try leftover chicken in a stir-fry or over a garden salad, or to make chicken chili. Remember, throwing away food is throwing away your money!

10 eating out
Restaurants can be expensive. Save money by getting the early bird special, going out for lunch instead of dinner, or looking for "2 for 1" deals. Stick to water instead of ordering other beverages, which add to the bill.

USDA
United States
Department of Agriculture
Center for Nutrition
Policy and Promotion

Go to www.ChooseMyPlate.gov for more information.

DG TipSheet No. 16
December 2011
USDA is an equal opportunity
provider and employer.

Today's Date: _____

Eating Healthy on a Budget Evaluation

1=Strongly Disagree	2=Disagree	3=Neither Disagree or Agree		4=Agree		5=Strongly Agree

	1	2	3	4	5
1. The workshop covered useful information. Comments:	1	2	3	4	5
2. The workshop activities were helpful. Comments:	1	2	3	4	5
3. I plan to plan meals for the week ahead of time this week. Comments:	1	2	3	4	5
4. I plan to change my eating habits based on the information I learned today. Comments:	1	2	3	4	5
5. I plan to become more active based on the information I learned today. Comments:	1	2	3	4	5
6. The instructor presented the information in a helpful way. Comments:	1	2	3	4	5
7. Overall, I found the workshop to be very helpful. Comments:	1	2	3	4	5

8. Please tell us which materials you found most useful.
Comments:

Workshop 4

Tips for Losing Weight and Keeping It Off

Eat Healthy ● *Be Active*
Community Workshops

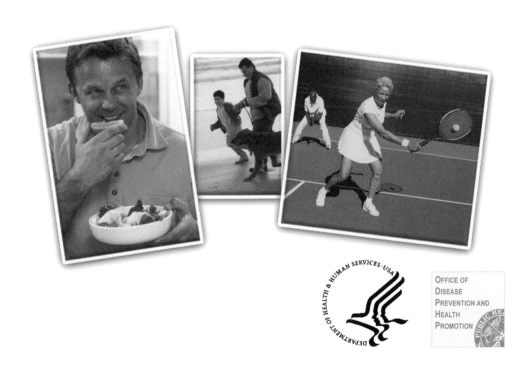

Instructor Guide

Before Workshop Begins

- Thoroughly read entire workshop and become familiar with the lesson plan.

- Gather materials needed for the icebreaker and activity.

  – *Icebreaker:* Various vegetables and fruits, cutting board, knife, plate/serving tray for vegetables/fruits, toothpicks. You also can make signs that list the name of each vegetable/fruit and what types of dishes you could make with it.

  Note: Wash and cut up the fruits/vegetables into bite-sized portions prior to class and put toothpicks in each for easy tasting.

  – *Activity:* Copies of *Rethink Your Drink* handout, pens/pencils

- Photocopy handouts (one per participant):

  1. Your Healthy Weight (1 page)

  2. Daily Calorie Needs (1 page)

  3. Top 4 Tips for Losing Weight and Keeping It Off (2 pages)

  4. "Rethink Your Drink" Matching Game (1 page)

  5. Calorie Log (3 pages)

  6. MyPlate/10 Tips to Use SuperTracker Your Way (2 pages)

  7. Workshop Evaluation (1 page)

Workshop Outline

The workshop should last ~1 hour, including activities.

- Icebreaker activity (5 minutes)—do this while people are coming into the workshop

- Introduction (5 minutes)

  – Explain the purpose of the workshop

  – Review the Learning Objectives

- **Objective 1:** Learn how to determine your body mass index (BMI) (5 minutes)
  - Review handout: *Your Healthy Weight* (help participants figure out their own BMI)

- **Objective 2:** Learn about the amount of calories you need each day (5 minutes)
  - Review handout: *Daily Calorie Needs*

- Stretch Break (5 minutes)

- **Objective 3:** Learn tips for losing weight and keeping it off (10–15 minutes)
  - Review handout: *Top 4 Tips for Losing Weight and Keeping It Off*
  - Review handout: *Calorie Log*

- Activity: Rethink Your Drink (5–10 minutes), using handout

- Review handout *MyPlate* and how to use *10 Tips to Use SuperTracker Your Way* (2 minutes)

- Wrap-up/Q&A (5–10 minutes)
  - Reminders of things to try at home:
    - Keep track of everything you eat and drink for 3 days this week
    - Slowly build up the amount of physical activity you do this week

- Ask participants to complete the evaluation form (5 minutes)

Workshop Lesson Plan

Icebreaker Activity—Taste Testing (5 minutes)

Fruits and Vegetables Tasting: Gather a variety of different fruits and vegetables (try items that may be unfamiliar to your population such as kiwi, jicama, papaya, passion fruit, okra, pomegranate, parsnip, etc.), and have participants taste a few as they come into the workshop.

Check out the Centers for Disease Control and Prevention's Fruit and Vegetable of the Month Web site for creative ideas of foods try: http://www.fruitsandveggiesmatter.gov/month/index.html

Note: Wash and cut up the fruits/vegetables into bite-sized portions prior to class and put toothpicks in each for easy tasting.

Supplies necessary: Various vegetables and fruits, cutting board, knife, plate/serving tray for vegetables/fruits, toothpicks. You also can make signs that list the name of each vegetable/fruit and what types of dishes you could make with it.

Talking Points—Purpose of the Workshop (2–3 minutes)

- Today's workshop and handouts will give you tips for losing weight and maintaining a healthy weight.

- This workshop is based on the *Dietary Guidelines for Americans, 2010* and the *2008 Physical Activity Guidelines for Americans*. The Dietary Guidelines provide science-based advice for making food choices that promote good health and a healthy weight and help prevent disease. The Physical Activity Guidelines provide recommendations on the amount, types, and level of intensity of physical activity needed to achieve and maintain good health.

- The Dietary Guidelines provide these selected consumer messages. More information about the messages can be found at http://www.ChooseMyPlate.gov.
  - *Balancing Calories*
    - ✓ Enjoy your food, but eat less.
    - ✓ Avoid oversized portions.
  - *Foods to Increase*
    - ✓ Make half your plate fruits and vegetables.

✓ Make at least half your grains whole grains.

✓ Switch to fat-free or low-fat (1%) milk.

– *Foods to Decrease*

✓ Compare sodium in foods like soup, bread, and frozen meals—and choose foods with lower numbers.

✓ Drink water instead of sugary drinks.

– Healthy eating and physical activity work hand in hand to help us live healthier lives. The Physical Activity Guidelines recommend that adults be physically active for at least 2 hours and 30 minutes each week—children need 60 minutes each day.

✓ You can stay physically active by doing activities such as walking, dancing, bicycling, or gardening and by reducing the amount of time you spend sitting.

Talking Points—Learning Objectives (2–3 minutes)

1. Learn how to determine your body mass index (BMI).

2. Learn about the amount of calories you need each day.

3. Learn tips for losing weight and keeping it off.

Talking Points—Handout: Your Healthy Weight (5 minutes)

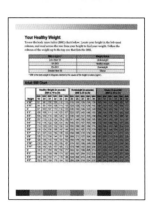

- BMI is a measure of your weight compared to your height. BMI can help adults determine whether they are at a healthy weight.

- BMI calculations don't work as well for people who are extremely muscular, very tall, or very short.

- Overall, BMI is a good indication of healthy weight for the majority of the adult population.

- BMI does not measure body fat. BMI is a quick and easy measure that can give you an idea of your weight status. Research has shown that BMI is often similar to body fat levels.

- Overweight or obese individuals are at increased risk for many diseases, such as: heart disease, high blood pressure, high cholesterol, type-2 diabetes, and some types of cancer.

- Additional information on BMI can be found here:
  http://www.cdc.gov/healthyweight/assessing/bmi/adult_bmi/index.html

Quick Activity: Determine Your BMI: Using the chart, help participants find the BMI for a man who weighs 218 pounds and is 5 feet 9 inches tall (answer: his BMI is 32, which is considered obese). Ask participants to determine their own BMI and what weight category they are in. *Note:* BMI can be a sensitive subject for participants and this is not something they need to share with the group.

Talking Points—Handout: Daily Calorie Needs (5 minutes)

- This chart shows how many calories are recommended for males and females in all age groups.

- You may need more or fewer calories depending on how active you are.

- If you want to lose weight, you will need to decrease the number of calories you eat each day and/or increase the amount of physical activity you do.

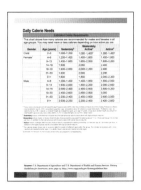

Stretch Break (5 minutes)

Muscle-strengthening activities provide additional benefits not found with aerobic activity. The benefits of muscle-strengthening activity include increased bone strength and muscular fitness. Muscle-strengthening activities also can help maintain muscle mass during a program of weight loss. Activities count as muscle-strengthening if they involve a moderate to high level of intensity or effort and work the major muscle groups of the body: the legs, hips, back, chest, abdomen, shoulders, and arms. Muscle-strengthening activities for all the major muscle groups should be done at least 2 days a week.

Ask each participant to do 5 repetitions of each exercise. You can repeat these two exercises 2 or 3 times, depending on time.

Standing Pushups (ask participants to spread out so each is facing a wall). Instructions: To begin, start standing up facing a wall. Place the palms of your hands on the wall at shoulder width apart with your arms fully extended. Press your body toward the wall so that your chest comes toward the wall and your elbows bend out to your sides (don't move your feet). Slowly press your body back to the starting position.

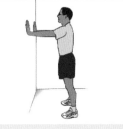

Modification: Stand closer to the wall so that your arms are not fully extended when you are doing the pushups.

Standing Squats (ask participants to stand up, with their feet shoulder width apart).

Instructions: Extend arms in front of your body. Keeping your weight on your heels, bend your knees and lower your hips down as if you were sitting in an imaginary "chair." Keep a neutral back and do not let your knees go past your toes.

Modification: Start sitting in a chair. Slowly stand up. Try not to use your arms and then slowly sit back in the chair (again, try not to use your arms).

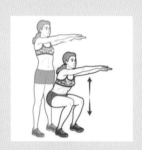

Talking Points—Handout: Top 4 Tips for Losing Weight and Keeping It Off (5–10 minutes)

- Reaching and maintaining a healthy weight is important for your overall health and well-being.

- If you are significantly overweight, you have a greater risk of developing many diseases or conditions, including high blood pressure, type-2 diabetes, stroke, and some forms of cancer.

- For obese adults, even losing a few pounds (such as 5-10% of your body weight) or preventing further weight gain has health benefits.

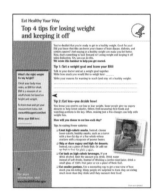

- Consuming fewer calories than expended will result in weight loss. This can be achieved over time by eating fewer calories, being more physically active, or, best of all, a combination of the two.

Learn Your BMI and Set a Weight Goal

- You just learned how to determine your BMI and your weight status category.

- A weight goal needs to be reasonable. If you want to lose weight, start with a goal of 5–10% of your current weight. For example, if you weigh 150 pounds, that would mean losing about 7–15 pounds. Make sure to talk to your doctor as well.

Eat Less

- Calorie balance over time is the key to weight management.

- Eat smaller portions. Try using smaller plates for dinner.

- Choose low-calorie snacks. Try foods such as fruits, vegetables, air-popped popcorn, fat-free yogurt, hummus, and almonds.

- Watch your intake of sugary and high-fat desserts—they can add a lot of extra calories and fats.

- Limit foods high in solid fats, such as butter/stick margarine, regular cheese, fatty meats, and French fries fried in oil.

- Drink more water and fat-free or low-fat (1%) milk and less regular soda, sports drinks, energy drinks, and fruit drinks.

Keep Track of What You Are Eating

- Keep track of what you eat for 3 or more days (using the *Calorie Log* handout or online at http://www.ChooseMyPlate.gov/supertracker) to get an idea of how many calories you are eating and drinking each day.

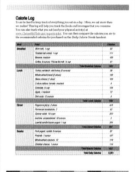

- The amount of calories you need varies depending on how active you are. See the *Daily Calorie Needs* handout to learn about your body's estimated calorie requirements.

- Weighing yourself regularly can help you determine whether you are eating the amount of calories that your body needs. If your weight is going up, cutting back on the amount of calories you are eating each day can help you lose weight.

Add Activity Every Day

- The *Physical Activity Guidelines for Americans* recommend that everyone engage in regular physical activity for health benefits.

- Here are the recommendations for adults:

	Moderate Activity	**Vigorous Activity**
Types of Activity	Walking briskly, biking on flat ground, line dancing, gardening	Jumping rope, basketball, soccer, swimming laps, aerobic dance
Amount	If you choose activities at a **moderate** level, do at least **2 hours and 30 minutes a week**	If you choose activities at a **vigorous** level, do at least **1 hour and 15 minutes a week**

- You can combine moderate and vigorous activities. In general, 1 minute of vigorous activity is equal to 2 minutes of moderate activity.

- Children need **60 minutes of physical activity each day.**

- **TODAY'S TIP:** Avoid inactivity.

  ✓ Every bit counts, and doing something is better than doing nothing!

  ✓ Start with a 10-minute chunk of physical activity a couple of days a week.

  ✓ Do a little more each time. Once you feel comfortable, do it more often. Then you can trade activities at a moderate level for vigorous ones that take more effort. You can do moderate and vigorous activities in the same week.

  ✓ Walking is one way to add physical activity to your life.

    – Build up to walking longer and more often.

    – Pick up the pace as you go.

- Consider signing up for the Presidential Active Lifestyle Award (PALA+) to help you track your physical activity and take small steps to improve your eating habits.

- If you are active for 30 minutes a day, 5 days a week for 6 out of 8 weeks, and choose one healthy eating goal each week to work toward, you'll be awarded the PALA+ and receive Presidential recognition! (See http://www.presidentschallenge.org) See handout in Appendix for more information.

Activity—Handout: "Rethink Your Drink" Matching Game (5–10 minutes)

"Rethink Your Drink" Matching Game: Ask participants to work with a partner and, using the worksheet, match the beverage with the number of calories. Using the answer key, go over answers with the group and discuss the better choices.

Supplies necessary: Copies of *Rethink Your Drink* handout, pens/pencils

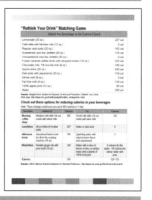

Talking Points—Activity: "Rethink Your Drink" Matching Game

- 100 calories can make a BIG difference. If you eat 100 calories less each day, over the course of 1 year, you could lose up to 10 pounds. 100 calories × 365 days = 365,000 calories/3,500 (number of calories in a pound) = approximately 10 lbs.

- An easy way to cut calories is from snacks and beverages. This activity shows how some beverages can be very high in calories.

- Instead of filling up on high-calorie beverages, think of your snacks as ways to get in more fruits and vegetables. Foods with fiber (whole-grain foods) and protein can help fill you up.

Answer Key for Activity

Beverage Calorie Count			
Lemonade (20 oz.)	280 cal.	Sports drink (20 oz.)	165 cal.
Café latte with fat-free milk (12 oz.)	125 cal.	Diet soda with aspartame (20 oz.)	0 cal.
Regular cola soda (20 oz.)	227 cal.	Whole milk (8 oz.)	150 cal.
Sweetened iced tea, bottled (20 oz.)	225 cal.	Fat-free milk (8 oz.)	90 cal.
Unsweetened iced tea, bottled (20 oz.)	3 cal.	100% apple juice (12 oz.)	192 cal.
Frozen caramel coffee drink with whipped cream (16 oz.)	430 cal.	Water	0 cal.
Chocolate milk, 1% low-fat milk (8 oz.)	158 cal.		

Talking Points—Handouts: MyPlate and 10 Tips (2 minutes)

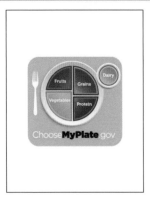
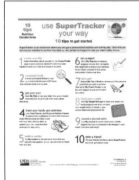

Talking Points—Wrap-up/Q&A (5 minutes)

Things to Try at Home

- Keep track of everything you eat and drink for 3 days this week.
- Continue to build up the amount of physical activity you choose to do.

Complete Evaluation Form (5 minutes)

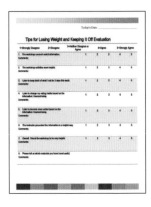

Workshop 4 ● Handouts

Your Healthy Weight

To use the body mass index (BMI) chart below: Locate your height in the left-most column, and read across the row from your height to find your weight. Follow the column of the weight up to the top row that lists the BMI.

BMI (in kg/m²)*	Weight Status
Less than 19	Underweight
19–24.9	Healthy weight
25–29.9	Overweight
Greater than 30	Obese

* BMI is the body weight in kilograms divided by the square of the height in meters (kg/m²).

Adult BMI Chart

Height	Healthy Weight (in pounds) (BMI is 19 to 24)						Overweight (in pounds) (BMI is 25 to 29)					Obese (in pounds) (BMI is 30 to 35)					
	BMI 19	BMI 20	BMI 21	BMI 22	BMI 23	BMI 24	BMI 25	BMI 26	BMI 27	BMI 28	BMI 29	BMI 30	BMI 31	BMI 32	BMI 33	BMI 34	BMI 35
4'10"	91	96	100	105	110	115	119	124	129	134	138	143	148	153	158	162	167
4'11"	94	99	104	109	114	119	124	128	133	138	143	148	153	158	163	168	173
5'	97	102	107	112	118	123	128	133	138	143	148	153	158	163	168	174	179
5'1"	100	106	111	116	122	127	132	137	143	148	153	158	164	169	174	180	185
5'2"	104	109	115	120	126	131	136	142	147	153	158	164	169	175	180	186	191
5'3"	107	113	118	124	130	135	141	146	152	158	163	169	175	180	186	191	197
5'4"	110	116	122	128	134	140	145	151	157	163	169	174	180	186	192	197	204
5'5"	114	120	126	132	138	144	150	156	162	168	174	180	186	192	198	204	210
5'6"	118	124	130	136	142	148	155	161	167	173	179	186	192	198	204	210	216
5'7"	121	127	134	140	146	153	159	166	172	178	185	191	198	204	211	217	223
5'8"	125	131	138	144	151	158	164	171	177	184	190	197	203	210	216	223	230
5'9"	128	135	142	149	155	162	169	176	182	189	196	203	209	216	223	230	236
5'10"	132	139	146	153	160	167	174	181	188	195	202	209	216	222	229	236	243
5'11"	136	143	150	157	165	172	179	186	193	200	208	215	222	229	236	243	250
6'	140	147	154	162	169	177	184	191	199	206	213	221	228	235	242	250	298
6'1"	144	151	159	166	174	182	189	197	204	212	219	227	235	242	250	257	265
6'2"	148	155	163	171	179	186	194	202	210	218	225	233	241	249	256	264	272
6'3"	152	160	168	176	184	192	200	208	216	224	232	240	248	256	264	272	279

Daily Calorie Needs

Estimated Calorie Requirements[a]

This chart shows how many calories are recommended for males and females in all age groups. You may need more or less calories depending on how active you are.

Gender	Age (years)	Sedentary[b]	Moderately Active[c]	Active[d]
Child	2–3	1,000–1,200	1,000–1,400[e]	1,000–1,400[e]
Female[f]	4–8	1,200–1,400	1,400–1,600	1,400–1,800
	9–13	1,400–1,600	1,600–2,000	1,800–2,200
	14–18	1,800	2,000	2,400
	19–30	1,800–2,000	2,000–2,200	2,400
	31–50	1,800	2,000	2,200
	51+	1,600	1,800	2,000–2,200
Male	4–8	1,200–1,400	1,400–1,600	1,600–2,000
	9–13	1,600–2,000	1,800–2,200	2,000–2,600
	14–18	2,000–2,400	2,400–2,800	2,800–3,200
	19–30	2,400–2,600	2,600–2,800	3,000
	31–50	2,200–2,400	2,400–2,600	2,800–3,000
	51+	2,000–2,200	2,200–2,400	2,400–2,800

[a] These levels are based on Estimated Energy Requirements (EER) from the Institute of Medicine (IOM) Dietary Reference Intakes macronutrients report, 2002, calculated by gender, age, and activity level for reference-sized individuals. "Reference size," as determined by IOM, is based on median height and weight for ages up to age 18 years of age and median height and weight for that height to give a body mass index (BMI) of 21.5 for adult females and 22.5 for adult males.

[b] **Sedentary** means a lifestyle that includes only the light physical activity associated with typical day-to-day life.

[c] **Moderately** active means a lifestyle that includes physical activity equivalent to walking about 1.5 to 3 miles per day at 3 to 4 miles per hour, in addition to the light physical activity associated with typical day-to-day life.

[d] **Active** means a lifestyle that includes physical activity equivalent to walking more than 3 miles per day at 3 to 4 miles per hour, in addition to the light physical activity associated with typical day-to-day life.

[e] The calorie ranges shown are to accommodate the needs of different ages within the group. For children and adolescents, more calories are needed at older ages. For adults, fewer calories are needed at older ages.

[f] Estimates for females do not include women who are pregnant or breastfeeding.

Source: U.S. Department of Agriculture and U.S. Department of Health and Human Services. *Dietary Guidelines for Americans, 2010*, page 14. http://www.cnpp.usda.gov/dietaryguidelines.htm

Top 4 tips for losing weight and keeping it off

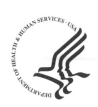

You've decided that you're ready to get to a healthy weight. Good for you! Did you know that this can lower your chance of heart disease, diabetes, and certain cancers? And staying at a healthy weight can make you feel better. Now, that's something to look forward to! Losing weight and keeping it off takes dedication. Yet, you can do this.
We wrote this handout to help you get started.

Tip 1: Set a weight goal and learn your BMI

Talk to your doctor and set a weight goal together.
Write how much you would like to weigh here: _____

Write your reasons for wanting to reach (and stay at) a healthy weight:

_____

_____

_____

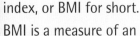

Tip 2: Eat less—you decide how!

You know you need to eat less to lose weight. Some people give up sugary desserts to help lower calories. Others find measuring their foods and watching portions is the key. Often, making just a few changes can help with weight loss.

How will you choose to eat less each day?

Tips to eating fewer calories:

- ❏ **Limit high-calorie snacks.** Instead, choose lower calorie, healthy snacks, such as a carrot with a low-fat dip or a few whole-wheat crackers with a teaspoon of peanut butter.

- ❏ **Skip or share sugary and high-fat desserts.** Instead, eat a piece of fresh fruit. Or add cut up fruit to low-fat plain yogurt.

- ❏ **Cut back on high-calorie beverages.** If you drink alcohol, limit the amount you drink. Drink water instead of soft drinks. Instead of drinking a jumbo-sized juice, drink a small glass of 100% fruit juice or eat a piece of fresh fruit.

- ❏ **Eat smaller portions.** Use a measuring cup to get a true view of how much you are eating. Many people are surprised to learn they are eating much more than they think until they measure their food!

What's the right weight for my height?

Check your body mass index, or BMI for short. BMI is a measure of an adult's body fat based on height and weight.

To learn more and get your measurement today, visit **www.nhlbisupport.com/bmi**

Write your BMI here:

_____

For more information, visit **www.healthfinder.gov**

(turn over please)

Small changes can make a large difference

Tip 3: Keep track of what you are eating

Studies show that tracking all your meals, snacks, and drinks can help weight loss. Keeping track will give you an idea of your eating patterns. It also can help you see areas where you are doing well and areas where you could improve. For example, are you snacking too much in the evening?

3 ways to track:

❑ Write down everything you eat and drink in a notebook.

❑ Track online at **www.choosemyplate.gov.**
Click "Assess Your Food Intake" to log what you eat and find out how well you're doing.

❑ Take a photo of the food with your cell phone to remind you of what you ate.

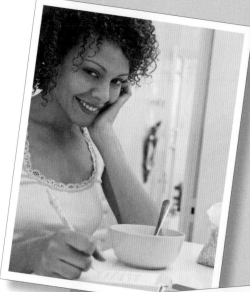

Tip 4: Add activity! It burns calories

Staying physically active can help you arrive and stay at a healthy weight. It makes sense—staying active helps you burn up some of the calories from foods. Most of us don't get enough activity to make up for what we eat.

Go to **www.choosemyplate.gov** to get tips on how you can stay active. You can also find out more about the types and amount of activity you need to get the most health benefits.

And remember, some physical activity is better than none!

Check off ways you can add activity into your day. Think of other things that you could do!

❑ Take the stairs　❑ Walk at lunch　❑ Hike with your kids

❑ Ride a bike　　　❑ Take up a sport　❑ Jog in place while watching TV

❑ Other ways to add activity to my day:

_____

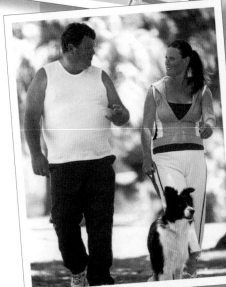

> **The key to staying at a healthy weight?
> Stay motivated!**
>
> Keep this sheet in a handy place to pull out to read now and again. Continue with your healthy eating and your physical activity habits. And bounce back if you get off your plan.

"Rethink Your Drink" Matching Game

Match the Beverage to Its Calorie Count	
Lemonade (20 oz.)	227 cal.
Café latte with fat-free milk (12 oz.)	3 cal.
Regular cola soda (20 oz.)	192 cal.
Sweetened iced tea, bottled (20 oz.)	125 cal.
Unsweetened iced tea, bottled (20 oz.)	0 cal.
Frozen caramel coffee drink with whipped cream (16 oz.)	225 cal.
Chocolate milk, 1% low-fat milk (8 oz.)	165 cal.
Sports drink (20 oz.)	430 cal.
Diet soda with aspartame (20 oz.)	158 cal.
Whole milk (8 oz.)	0 cal.
Fat-free milk (8 oz.)	150 cal.
100% apple juice (12 oz.)	90 cal.
Water	280 cal.

Source: Adapted from Centers for Disease Control and Prevention, Rethink Your Drink
Web page. http://www.cdc.gov/healthyweight/healthy_eating/drinks.html

Check out these options for reducing calories in your beverages

Note: These changes could save you up to 650 calories in 1 day!

Occasion	Instead of . . .	Calories	Try . . .	Calories
Morning coffee shop	Medium café latte (16 oz) made with whole milk	265	Small café latte (12 oz) made with skim milk	125
Lunchtime	20-oz bottle of nondiet soda	227	Water or diet soda	0
Afternoon break	Sweetened lemon iced tea from the vending machine (16 oz)	180	Sparkling water with natural lemon flavor (not sweetened)	0
Dinnertime	Nondiet ginger ale with your meal (12 oz)	124	Water with a slice of lemon or lime, or seltzer water with a splash of 100% fruit juice	0 calories for the water, ~30 calories for seltzer water with juice
Calories		796		125–155

Source: USDA National Nutrient Database for Standard Reference. http://www.nal.usda.gov/fnic/foodcomp/search/

Calorie Log

It can be hard to keep track of everything you eat in a day. Often, we eat more than we realize! This log will help you track the foods and beverages that you consume. You can also track what you eat (and your physical activity) at www.choosemyplate.gov/supertracker. You can then compare the calories you ate to the recommended calories for you based on the *Daily Calorie Needs* handout.

Meal	Food	Calories
Breakfast	[At home] Skim milk, 1 cup	83
	[At home] Toasted oat cereal, 1 cup	111
	[At home] Banana, medium	105
	[At home] Coffee, 8 ounces 1% low-fat milk, ½ cup	61
	Total Breakfast Calories	**360**
Lunch	[Office cafeteria] Turkey sandwich: deli turkey (2 ounces)	59
	[Office cafeteria] whole-wheat bread, Swiss cheese (1 slice)	130
	[Office cafeteria] 2 slices lettuce, tomato, mustard	114
	[Office cafeteria] Coleslaw, ½ cup	134
	[Office cafeteria] Apple, 1 medium	72
	[Office cafeteria] Diet soda, 12 ounces	0
	Total Lunch Calories	**509**
Dinner	[Restaurant] Pepperoni pizza, 2 slices	416
	[Restaurant] Parmesan breadsticks, 2	82
	[Restaurant] Caesar salad, 1½ cups	253
	[Restaurant] Iced tea, unsweetened, 16 ounces	5
	[Restaurant] Low-fat vanilla frozen yogurt, 1 cup	241
	Total Dinner Calories	**997**
Snacks	[Home, office] Fruit yogurt, nonfat, 8 ounces	87
	[Home, office] Pretzels, 1 ounce	107
	[Home, office] Whole-wheat crackers, 12	114
	[Home, office] Cheddar cheese, 1 ounce	114
	Total Snacks Calories	**422**
	Total Daily Calories	**2,261**

Day 1

Meal	Food	Calories
Breakfast		
	Total Breakfast Calories	
Lunch		
	Total Lunch Calories	
Dinner		
	Total Dinner Calories	
Snacks		
	Total Snacks Calories	
	Total Daily Calories	

Day 2

Meal	Food	Calories
Breakfast		
	Total Breakfast Calories	
Lunch		
	Total Lunch Calories	
Dinner		
	Total Dinner Calories	
Snacks		
	Total Snacks Calories	
	Total Daily Calories	

Day 3

Meal	Food	Calories
Breakfast		
	Total Breakfast Calories	
Lunch		
	Total Lunch Calories	
Dinner		
	Total Dinner Calories	
Snacks		
	Total Snacks Calories	
	Total Daily Calories	

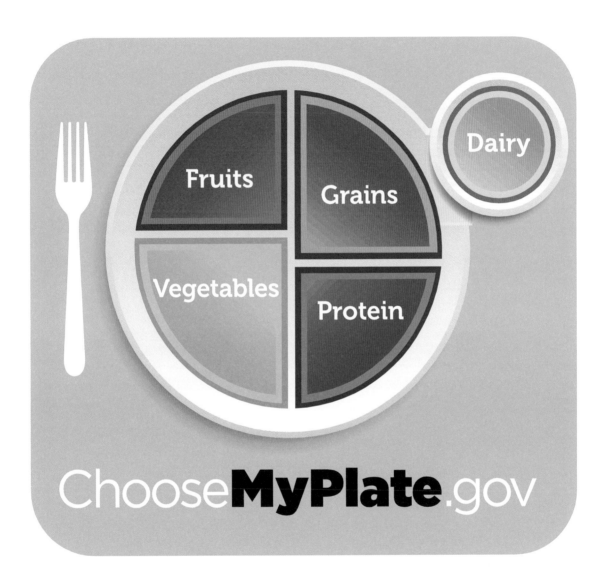

Choose MyPlate.gov

10 tips
Nutrition Education Series

use **SuperTracker** your way
10 **tips** to get started

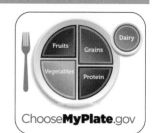
ChooseMyPlate.gov

SuperTracker is an online tool where you can get a personalized nutrition and activity plan. Track what you eat and your activities to see how they stack up, and get tips and support to help you make healthy choices.

1 create a profile
Enter information about yourself on the **Create Profile** page to get a personal calorie limit and food plan; register to save your data and access it any time.

2 compare foods
Check out **Food-A-Pedia** to look up nutrition info for over 8,000 foods and compare foods side by side.

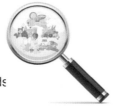

3 get your plan
View **My Plan** to see your daily food group targets— what and how much to eat within your calorie allowance.

4 track your foods and activities
Use **Food Tracker** and **Physical Activity Tracker** to search from a database of over 8,000 foods and nearly 800 physical activities to see how your daily choices stack up against your plan; save favorites and copy for easy entry.

5 build a combo
Try **My Combo** to link and save foods that you typically eat together, so you can add them to meals with one click.

6 run a report
Go to **My Reports** to measure progress; choose from six reports that range from a simple meal summary to an indepth analysis of food group and nutrient intakes over time.

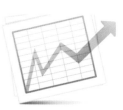

7 set a goal
Explore **My Top 5 Goals** to choose up to five personal goals that you want to achieve. Sign up for **My Coach Center** to get tips and support as you work toward your goals.

8 track your weight
Visit **My Weight Manager** to enter your weight and track progress over time; compare your weight history to trends in your calorie intake and physical activity.

9 record a journal entry
Use **My Journal** to record daily events; identify triggers that may be associated with changes in your health behaviors and weight.

10 refer a friend!
Tell your friends and family about **SuperTracker**; help them get started today.

USDA
United States Department of Agriculture
Center for Nutrition Policy and Promotion

DG TipSheet No. 17
December 2011
USDA is an equal opportunity provider and employer.

Go to www.ChooseMyPlate.gov for more information.

Tips for Losing Weight and Keeping It Off Evaluation

1=Strongly Disagree	2=Disagree	3=Neither Disagree or Agree	4=Agree	5=Strongly Agree

	1	2	3	4	5
1. The workshop covered useful information. Comments:	1	2	3	4	5
2. The workshop activities were helpful. Comments:	1	2	3	4	5
3. I plan to keep track of what I eat for 3 days this week. Comments:	1	2	3	4	5
4. I plan to change my eating habits based on the information I learned today. Comments:	1	2	3	4	5
5. I plan to become more active based on the information I learned today. Comments:	1	2	3	4	5
6. The instructor presented the information in a helpful way. Comments:	1	2	3	4	5
7. Overall, I found the workshop to be very helpful. Comments:	1	2	3	4	5

8. Please tell us which materials you found most useful.
Comments:

Workshop 5

Making Healthy Eating Part of Your Total Lifestyle

Eat Healthy ● *Be Active*
Community Workshops

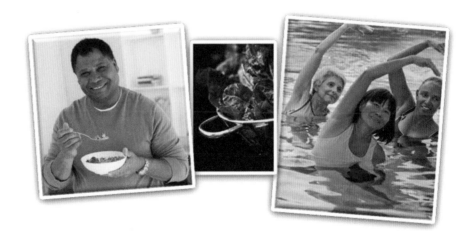

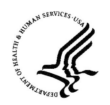

OFFICE OF
DISEASE
PREVENTION AND
HEALTH
PROMOTION

Instructor Guide

Before Workshop Begins

- Thoroughly read entire workshop and become familiar with the lesson plan.

- Gather materials needed for the icebreaker and activity.

  - *Icebreaker:* A variety of whole grain foods, such as whole wheat pasta (cooked prior to class), brown rice (cooked prior to class), whole wheat bread (cut into portions to try), whole grain crackers, whole grain cereal, etc., serving plates and utensils for participants to try foods offered.

  - *Activity:* No supplies necessary

- Photocopy handouts (one per participant):

  1. Making Healthy Eating Part of Your Total Lifestyle (2 pages)

  2. GO, SLOW, and WHOA Foods (2 pages)

  3. Tips for Using the Nutrition Facts Label (1 page)

  4. MyPlate/10 Tips to Enjoy Your Food, But Eat Less (2 pages)

  5. Workshop Evaluation (1 page)

Workshop Outline

The workshop should last ~1 hour, including activities.

- Icebreaker activity (5 minutes)—do this while people are coming into the workshop

- Introduction (5 minutes)

  - Explain the purpose of the workshop

  - Review the Learning Objectives

- **Objective 1:** Learn the concepts of a healthy lifestyle (10 minutes)

  - Review handout: *Making Healthy Eating Part of Your Total Lifestyle*

- Stretch Break (5 minutes)

- **Objective 2:** Learn about foods that should be eaten regularly and those that should be eaten only occasionally (5 minutes)

  - Review handout: *GO, SLOW, and WHOA Foods*

- **Objective 3:** Learn how to read and understand the Nutrition Facts Label (5 minutes)

- Activity (5–10 minutes)

  – Review handout: *Tips for Using the Nutrition Facts Label*

- Increasing Physical Activity (1–2 minutes)

- Review handout *MyPlate* and how to use *10 Tips to Enjoy Your Food, But Eat Less* (2 minutes)

- Wrap-up/Q&A (5 minutes)

  – Reminders of things to try at home:

    ■ Read the Nutrition Facts Labels to compare food at the grocery store

    ■ Continue to build up the amount of physical activity you do each day

- Ask participants to complete the evaluation form (5 minutes)

Workshop Lesson Plan

Icebreaker Activity—Taste Testing (5 minutes)

Whole Grain Tasting: Gather a variety of different whole grain foods (try items such as pasta, rice, cereal, crackers, bread, etc.) and have participants taste a few as they come into the workshop.

Supplies necessary: A variety of whole grain foods, such as whole wheat pasta (cooked prior to class), brown rice (cooked prior to class), whole wheat bread (cut into portions to try), whole grain crackers, whole grain cereal, etc., serving plates and utensils for participants to try foods selected.

Talking Points—Purpose of the Workshop (2–3 minutes)

- Today's workshop and handouts will give you tips for incorporating a healthy diet and regular physical activity into your lifestyle.

- This workshop is based on the *Dietary Guidelines for Americans, 2010* and the *2008 Physical Activity Guidelines for Americans*. The Dietary Guidelines provide science-based advice for making food choices that promote good health and a healthy weight and help prevent disease. The Physical Activity Guidelines provide recommendations on the amount, types, and level of intensity of physical activity needed to achieve and maintain good health.

- The Dietary Guidelines provide these selected consumer messages. More information about the messages can be found at http://www.ChooseMyPlate.gov.

  - *Balancing Calories*
    - ✓ Enjoy your food, but eat less.
    - ✓ Avoid oversized portions.

  - *Foods to Increase*
    - ✓ Make half your plate fruits and vegetables.
    - ✓ Make at least half your grains whole grains.
    - ✓ Switch to fat-free or low-fat (1%) milk.

  - *Foods to Decrease*
    - ✓ Compare sodium in foods like soup, bread, and frozen meals—and choose foods with lower numbers.
    - ✓ Drink water instead of sugary drinks.

– Healthy eating and physical activity work hand in hand to help us live healthier lives. The Physical Activity Guidelines recommend that adults be physically active for at least 2 hours and 30 minutes each week—children need 60 minutes each day.

✓ You can stay physically active by doing activities such as walking, dancing, bicycling, or gardening and by reducing the amount of time you spend sitting.

Talking Points—Learning Objectives (2–3 minutes)

1. Learn the concepts of a healthy lifestyle.

2. Learn about foods that should be eaten regularly and those that should be eaten only occasionally.

3. Learn how to read and understand the Nutrition Facts Label.

Talking Points—Handout: Making Healthy Eating Part of Your Total Lifestyle (10 minutes)

Note: These talking points cover all of the key consumer behaviors and potential strategies for professionals in the Dietary Guidelines. Depending on time/participant questions, you may choose to cover just a few bullets under each heading.

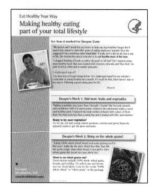

Add More Fruits and Vegetables

Vegetables

- Make half your plate vegetables and fruits, especially nutrient-packed ones that are red, orange, and green.

- Include vegetables in meals and in snacks. Fresh, frozen, and canned vegetables all count. When eating canned vegetables, choose those labeled as reduced sodium or no-salt-added.

- Add dark green, red, and orange vegetables to soups, stews, casseroles, stir-fries, and other main and side dishes. Use dark leafy greens, such as romaine lettuce and spinach, to make salads.

- Focus on dietary fiber—beans and peas are a great source. Add beans or peas to salads (e.g., kidney or garbanzo beans), soups (e.g., split peas or lentils), and side dishes (e.g., baked beans or pinto beans), or serve as a main dish.

- Keep raw, cut-up vegetables handy for quick snacks. If serving with a dip, choose lower calorie options, such as yogurt-based dressings or hummus, instead of sour cream or cream cheese-based dips.

- When eating out, choose a vegetable as a side dish. With cooked vegetables, request that they be prepared with little or no fat and salt. With salads, ask for the dressing on the side so you can decide how much you use.

- When adding sauces, condiments, or dressings to vegetables, use small amounts and look for lower calorie options (e.g., reduced-fat cheese sauce or fat-free dressing). Sauces can make vegetables more appealing, but often add extra calories.

Fruits

- Use fruit as snacks, salads, or desserts.

- Instead of sugars, syrups, or other sweet toppings, use fruit to top foods such as cereal and pancakes.

- Enjoy a wide variety of fruits, and maximize taste and freshness by adapting your choices to what is in season.

- Keep rinsed and cut-up fruit handy for quick snacks.

- Use canned, frozen, and dried fruits, as well as fresh fruits. Unsweetened fruit or fruit canned in 100% juice is the better choice because light or heavy syrup adds sugar and calories.

- Select 100% fruit juice when choosing juices.

Bring on the Whole Grains

- Substitute whole-grain choices for refined grains in breakfast cereals, breads, crackers, rice, and pasta.

- For example, choose 100% whole-grain breads; whole-grain cereals such as oatmeal; whole-grain crackers and pasta; and brown rice. Check the ingredients list on product labels for the words "whole" or "whole-grain" before the grain ingredient's name.

- Note that foods labeled with the words "multi-grain," "stone-ground," "100% wheat," "cracked wheat," "seven-grain," or "bran" are usually not 100% whole-grain products, and may not contain any whole grains.

- Use the Nutrition Facts Label and the ingredients list to choose whole grains that are a good or excellent source of dietary fiber.

- Good sources of fiber contain 10–19% of the Daily Value per serving, and excellent sources of dietary fiber contain 20% or more.

Cut Back on Sodium and Salt

- Use the Nutrition Facts Label to choose foods lower in sodium.

- When purchasing canned foods, select those labeled as "reduced sodium," "low sodium" or " no salt added." Rinse regular canned foods to remove some sodium. Many packaged foods contain more sodium than their made-from-fresh counterparts.

- Use little or no salt when cooking or eating. Trade in your salt shaker for a pepper shaker. Spices, herbs, and lemon juice can be used as alternatives to salt to season foods with a variety of flavors.

- Gradually reduce the amount of sodium in your foods. Your taste for salt will change over time.

- Get more potassium in your diet. Food sources of potassium include potatoes, cantaloupe, bananas, beans, and yogurt.

Putting It All Together

- Start by making small changes and eating a variety of foods that your body needs for good health.

Stretch Break (5 minutes)

"Fruit Basket"—a nutrition-themed version of musical chairs

This is a simple game that's best for a group of at least eight players. Set up a circle with enough chairs for all of your players minus one. Next, you'll need to assign each player a fruit, labeling players as *strawberry, orange, banana*, etc. Two players should be assigned to each fruit. One person should remain standing, and everyone else should sit in the chairs. The standing person will call out a fruit name, and any player sitting in the circle assigned to that fruit then has to jump up and try to find a new seat. The caller also should try as fast as possible to sit in one of the open seats. In the end, a player will be left without a seat. That player (left standing) will then call out another fruit, and the game continues. For fun, try calling out more than one fruit at a time. The caller also has the option of calling out "fruit basket!" When that happens, *all* players get up from their chairs and find a new one. It gets a little crazy as everyone tries to get a seat. If needed, you can set a rule that a player getting up from a chair must find a new one at least two seats away (to encourage players to get up and run around).

Talking Points—Handout: GO, SLOW, and WHOA Foods (5 minutes)

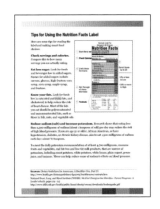

- **GO** foods contain a low amount of fat and added sugar. They are rich in nutrients and relatively low in calories. Examples of **GO** foods include fruits and vegetables, whole-grain foods without added fats, fat-free or low-fat (1%) milk and milk products, and lean cuts of meat. Enjoy **GO** foods almost any time.

- **SLOW** foods are higher in fat and added sugar than **GO** foods. Examples of **SLOW** foods include vegetables prepared with added fat (such as butter) and sauces, French toast, fruit canned in syrup, and 2% low-fat milk. Have **SLOW** foods sometimes or less often.

- **WHOA** foods are the highest in fat and added sugar of the three groups. **WHOA** foods have the most calories, and many are low in nutrients. Examples of **WHOA** foods include fried foods; baked goods such as croissants, doughnuts, cakes, and pies; whole milk; candy; regular soda; and chips. Have **WHOA** foods only once in a while or on special occasions.

Activity—Using a Nutrition Facts Label (5–10 minutes)

Nutrition Facts Label: Pass out handout *Tips for Reading the Nutrition Facts Label* and review the talking points listed below. Depending on the size of the group, you may want to pass out a label for each group of 2–3 people to work together to identify components of the food label, such as portion size, sodium, etc.

Supplies necessary: A variety of nutrition facts labels from food containers.

Talking Points—Handout: Tips for Using the Nutrition Facts Label (5 minutes)

- Look at the serving size and determine how many servings you are actually eating.

  - If you eat two servings of a food, you will consume double the calories.

- Choose foods with less sugar.

  - Foods with added sugars (names include sucrose, glucose, high fructose corn syrup, corn syrup, maple syrup, and fructose) provide calories with few nutrients. Make sure that added sugars are not one of the first few ingredients.

- Look for foods low in solid fats (saturated and *trans* fat) and cholesterol to help reduce the risk of heart disease. Choose healthier fats, such as polyunsaturated and monounsaturated fats, found in fish, nuts, and vegetable oils.

- Compare sodium in products. Most sodium comes from processed foods.

  – A diet rich in potassium can help reverse some of the effects of sodium on blood pressure.

Talking Points—Increasing Physical Activity (1–2 minutes)

- The *Physical Activity Guidelines for Americans* recommend that everyone engage in regular physical activity for health benefits.

- Here are the recommendations for adults:

	Moderate Activity	Vigorous Activity
Types of Activity	Walking briskly, biking on flat ground, line dancing, gardening	Jumping rope, basketball, soccer, swimming laps, aerobic dance
Amount	If you choose activities at a moderate level, do at least **2 hours and 30 minutes a week**	If you choose activities at a vigorous level, do at least **1 hour and 15 minutes a week**

- You can combine moderate and vigorous activities. In general, 1 minute of vigorous activity is equal to 2 minutes of moderate activity.

- Children need **60 minutes of physical activity each day.**

- **TODAY'S TIP:** Slowly build up the amount of physical activity you choose.

  ✓ Start with 10 minutes of activity, and then add time so you are being active for longer each time.

  ✓ As you feel more comfortable, do more by being active more often and increasing the pace of your activity.

- Consider signing up for the Presidential Active Lifestyle Award (PALA+) to help you track your physical activity and take small steps to improve your eating habits.

- If you are active for 30 minutes a day, 5 days a week for 6 out of 8 weeks, and choose one nutrition goal each week to work toward, you'll be awarded the PALA+ and receive Presidential recognition! (See http://www.presidentschallenge.org) See handout in Appendix for more information.

Talking Points—Handouts: MyPlate and 10 Tips (2 minutes)

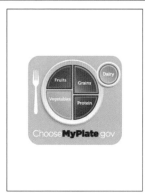
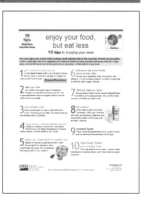

Talking Points—Wrap-up/Q&A (5 minutes)

Things to Try at Home

- Read the Nutrition Facts Labels to compare food at the grocery store.
- Slowly build up the amount of physical activity you do each day.

Complete Evaluation Form (5 minutes)

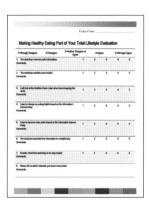

Workshop 5 ● Handouts

Eat Healthy Your Way
Making healthy eating part of your total lifestyle

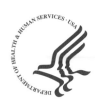

See how it worked for Dwayne Davis

"My doctor said I needed to eat better to help me stay healthier longer. But I wasn't sure where to start after years of eating whatever I wanted. Then she suggested I try something called **'total diet.'** It really isn't a diet at all—but a way of life. The bottom line about total diet is to **eat healthy most of the time.**

"I stopped thinking of foods as either 'all good' or 'all bad.' First I started eating more healthy foods that were loaded with vitamins, minerals, and fiber. And I ate junk food less often and in smaller amounts."

I challenged myself!

"I've done lots of tough things before. So I challenged myself to see whether I could stick to eating healthy for a month. If I could do that, then I knew I was on my way to following a good eating plan for life."

Dwayne

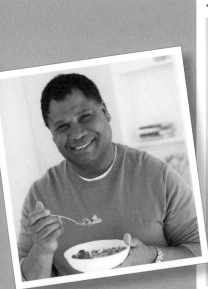

Dwayne's Week 1: Add more fruits and vegetables

"Adding vegetables was easier than I thought. I found I like broccoli, spinach, and cauliflower. Half of a sweet potato cooked in the microwave makes a sweet and healthy snack. I replaced my usual cookies at lunch with a piece of fresh fruit. The fruit costs less than a candy bar and is loaded with fiber and vitamins."

Ready to try more vegetables?
Go for the red and orange (sweet potatoes, carrots) and green (broccoli, spinach) kinds to get the most nutrients.

Dwayne's Week 2: Bring on the whole grains!

"Eating 100% whole-wheat bread took some getting used to. But now I really like the taste. And it has fiber that fills me up for longer than white bread. I even prefer other whole grains like brown rice over white rice."

Want to eat whole grains too?
Good choices include 100% whole-wheat pasta, breads, and tortillas. Try rolled oats and brown rice too. Read labels. Look for the words "100% whole wheat" or "whole grain" on the package.

▼
For more information, visit www.healthfinder.gov

(turn over please)

Small changes can make a large difference

Dwayne's Week 3: Cut back on salt (sodium) and sugar

"Once I started reading labels, I was surprised at how much sodium is in packaged foods. High blood pressure runs in my family and cutting back on salt makes a lot of sense health-wise. And sugar? I stopped drinking my daily super-sized 64-ounce soft drink. Turned out the drink had 800 calories—about half of what many people need for the whole day!"

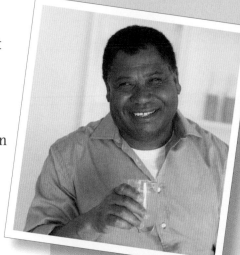

Limit how often and how much salt you eat.

Eat less of these salty foods: pickles, soy sauce, hot dogs, lunch meats, chips, and pretzels. Look for the words "low sodium" or "no salt added" on **canned** vegetables, vegetable juices, and soups.

Eat fewer sweets.

Cut back on empty calories that offer you no nutrients. Eat fruit instead of desserts. Drink fat-free milk, water, or a small glass of 100% juice instead of sugary soft drinks.

From Week 4 on: Put it all together for a successful healthy eating plan

"By making small changes over time I was beginning to follow a healthy food plan I knew I could stick to. And you know what? I felt better **and** I also lost weight."

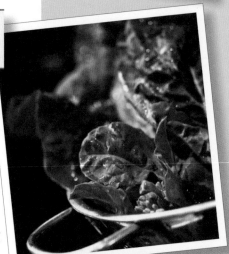

Food experts suggest eating a variety of foods that give you what your body needs for good health. No food is forbidden—the key is to eat far more of the foods that are good for you and less of the foods that aren't.

The bottom line?
Watch how much you eat of each food. For more about portion and serving sizes, visit **www.win.niddk.nih.gov/publications/just_enough.htm**.

Include these foods in your food plan:

- ❑ Fruits and vegetables.
- ❑ Whole grains, such as brown rice, oats, whole-wheat pasta, and whole-grain breads.
- ❑ Foods with a lot of calcium, such as fat-free milk and milk products like low-fat yogurt and reduced-fat cheese. Spinach, collard greens, and kale are a source of calcium.
- ❑ Lean meats, light meat chicken and turkey, fish, eggs, and beans.
- ❑ Healthy fats, such as olive oil, canola oil, and nuts. Just watch your portions.

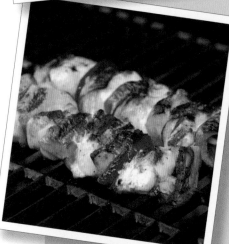

Now that you've read Dwayne's story . . .
What tips will you try as you follow a healthy total diet?

ODPHP Publication No. U0053

GO, SLOW, and WHOA Foods

Use this chart as a guide to help you and your family make smart food choices. Post it on your refrigerator at home, or take it with you to the store when you shop.

GO foods—Eat almost anytime.
SLOW foods—Eat sometimes or less often.
WHOA foods—Eat only once in a while or for special occasions.

Food Group	GO Almost anytime foods (Nutrient-dense foods)	SLOW Sometimes foods (Moderate nutrients/calories)	WHOA Once in a while foods (Calorie dense foods)
Vegetables	Almost all fresh, frozen, and canned vegetables without added fat and sauces	All vegetables with added fat and sauces; oven-baked French fries; avocado	Fried potatoes, like French fries or hash browns; other deep-fried vegetables
Fruits	All fresh, frozen, canned in juice	100% fruit juice; fruits canned in light syrup; dried fruits	Fruits canned in heavy syrup
Breads and Cereals	Whole-grain breads, including pita bread; tortillas and whole-grain pasta; brown rice; hot and cold unsweetened whole-grain breakfast cereals	White refined flour bread, rice, and pasta; French toast; taco shells; cornbread; biscuits; granola; waffles and pancakes	Croissants; muffins; doughnuts; sweet rolls; crackers made with trans fats; calorically sweetened breakfast cereals
Milk and Milk Products	Fat-free or 1% low-fat milk; fat-free or low-fat yogurt; part skim, reduced-fat, and fat-free cheese; low-fat or fat-free cottage cheese	2% low-fat milk; processed cheese spread	Whole milk; full-fat American, cheddar, Colby, Swiss, or cream cheese; whole-milk yogurt
Meats, Poultry, Fish, Eggs, Beans, and Nuts	Trimmed beef and pork; extra-lean ground beef; chicken and turkey without skin; tuna canned in water; baked, broiled, steamed, or grilled fish and shellfish; beans, split peas, lentils, tofu; egg whites and egg substitutes	Lean ground beef; broiled hamburgers; ham, Canadian bacon; chicken and turkey with skin; low-fat hot dogs; tuna canned in oil; peanut butter; nuts; whole eggs cooked without added fat	Untrimmed beef and pork; regular ground beef; fried hamburgers; ribs; bacon; fried chicken, chicken nuggets; hot dogs, lunch meats, pepperoni, sausage; fried fish and shellfish; whole eggs cooked with fat
Sweets and Snacks*		Ice milk bars; frozen fruit juice bars; low-fat or fat-free frozen yogurt and ice-cream; fig bars, ginger snaps, baked chips; low-fat microwave popcorn; pretzels	Cookies and cakes; pies; cheesecake; ice cream; chocolate; candy; chips; buttered microwave popcorn

* Though some of the foods in this row are lower in fat and calories, all sweets and snacks need to be limited, in order to stay within one's daily calorie needs.

Food Group	GO Almost anytime foods (Nutrient-dense foods)	SLOW Sometimes foods (Moderate nutrients/calories)	WHOA Once in a while foods (Calorie dense foods)
Fats/ Condiments	Vinegar; ketchup; mustard; fat-free creamy salad dressing; fat-free mayonnaise; fat-free sour cream	Vegetable oil,** olive oil, and oil-based salad dressing; soft margarine; low-fat creamy salad dressing; low-fat mayonnaise; low-fat sour cream	Butter, stick margarine; lard; salt pork; gravy; regular creamy salad dressing; mayonnaise; tartar sauce; sour cream; cheese sauce; cream sauce; cream cheese dips
Beverages	Water, fat-free milk or 1% low-fat milk; diet soda; unsweetened iced tea or diet iced tea and lemonade	2% low-fat milk; 100% fruit juice; sports drinks	Whole milk; regular soda; calorically sweetened iced teas and lemonade; fruit drinks with less than 100% fruit juice

** Vegetable and olive oils contain no saturated or *trans* fats and can be consumed daily, but in limited portions to meet daily calorie needs.

How you choose to prepare or order your food when eating out can quickly turn a less healthy food into a healthier option. Choosing baked, broiled, steamed, grilled, and microwaved foods saves you from extra fat and calories. See the examples below on how similar foods can go from a GO to a SLOW or a WHOA food.

	GO (eat almost anytime)	Calories	SLOW (eat sometimes or less often)	Calories	WHOA (eat once in a while)	Calories
Fruit	Apple, 1 medium	72	Baked apple, 1 cup slices, with 1 Tbsp. butter	193	Apple pie, ⅛ of 9-inch pie	296
Bread	½ whole-wheat bagel (3½ inch)	91	½ plain bagel (3½ inch) with 1 Tbsp. jelly	147	½ plain bagel (3½ inch) with 1 Tbsp. butter and jelly	249
Meat	Roasted chicken breast without skin, ½ breast	142	Roasted chicken breast with skin, ½ breast	193	Fried chicken, 2 drumsticks	386

Source: Adapted from National Heart, Lung, and Blood Institute (NHLBI), *We Can! Energize Our Families—Parent Program: A Leader's Guide,* pages 116–117.
http://www.nhlbi.nih.gov/health/public/heart/obesity/wecan/downloads/leadersguide.pdf

Tips for Using the Nutrition Facts Label

Here are some tips for reading the label and making smart food choices:

Check servings and calories. Compare this to how many servings you are actually eating.

Eat less sugar. Look for foods and beverages low in added sugars. Names for added sugars include sucrose, glucose, high fructose corn syrup, corn syrup, maple syrup, and fructose.

Know your fats. Look for foods low in saturated and *trans* fats, and cholesterol, to help reduce the risk of heart disease. Most of the fats you eat should be polyunsaturated and monounsaturated fats, such as those in fish, nuts, and vegetable oils.

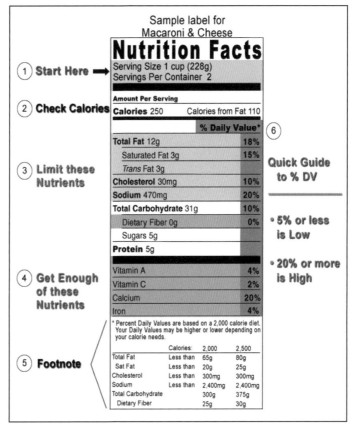

Reduce sodium (salt) and increase potassium. Research shows that eating less than 2,300 milligrams of sodium (about 1 teaspoon of salt) per day may reduce the risk of high blood pressure. If you are age 51 or older, African American, or have hypertension, diabetes, or chronic kidney disease, aim to eat 1,500 milligrams of sodium each day—about ¾ teaspoon.

To meet the daily potassium recommendation of at least 4,700 milligrams, consume fruits and vegetables, and fat-free and low-fat milk products, that are sources of potassium, including sweet potatoes, white potatoes, white beans, plain yogurt, prune juice, and bananas. These can help reduce some of sodium's effects on blood pressure.

Sources: Dietary Guidelines for Americans, *A Healthier You*, Part III.
http://www.health.gov/dietaryguidelines/dga2005/healthieryou/contents.htm

National Heart, Lung, and Blood Institute (NHLBI), **We Can!** *Energize Our Families—Parent Program: A Leader's Guide,* pages 114–115.
http://www.nhlbi.nih.gov/health/public/heart/obesity/wecan/downloads/leadersguide.pdf

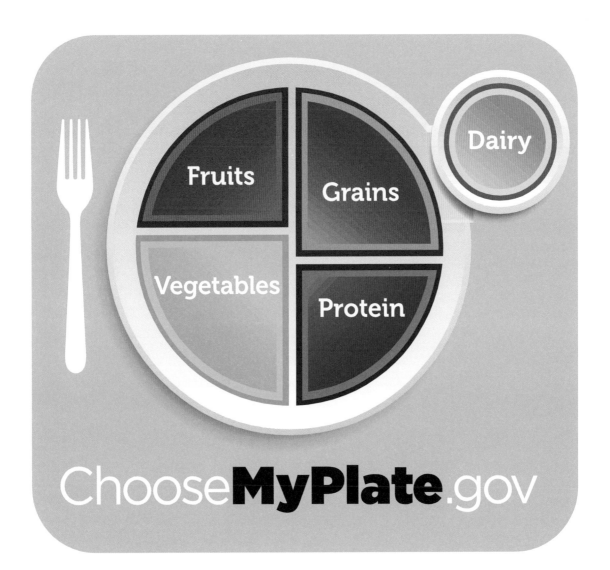

10 tips
Nutrition Education Series

enjoy your food, but eat less

10 **tips** to enjoying your meal

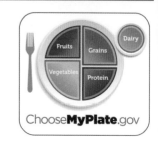
Choose**MyPlate**.gov

You can enjoy your meals while making small adjustments to the amounts of food on your plate. Healthy meals start with more vegetables and fruits and smaller portions of protein and grains. And don't forget dairy—include fat-free or low-fat dairy products on your plate, or drink milk with your meal.

1 get to know the foods you eat
Use the **SuperTracker** to find out what kinds of foods and how much to eat and to get tips and support for making better food choices.

SuperTracker

2 take your time
Be mindful to eat slowly, enjoy the taste and textures, and pay attention to how you feel. Use hunger and fullness cues to recognize when to eat and when you've had enough.

3 use a smaller plate
Use a smaller plate at meals to help with portion control. That way you can finish your entire plate and feel satisfied without overeating.

4 if you eat out, choose healthier options
Check and compare nutrition information about the foods you are eating. Preparing food at home makes it easier to control what is in your meals.

5 satisfy your sweet tooth in a healthy way
Indulge in a naturally sweet dessert dish—fruit! Serve a fresh fruit cocktail or a fruit parfait made with yogurt. For a hot dessert, bake apples and top with cinnamon.

6 choose to eat some foods more or less often
Choose more vegetables, fruits, whole grains, and fat-free or 1% milk and dairy products. Cut back on foods high in solid fats, added sugars, and salt.

7 find out what you need
Get your personalized plan by using the **SuperTracker** to identify your food group targets. Compare the foods you eat to the foods you need to eat.

8 sip smarter
Drink water or other calorie-free beverages, 100% juice, or fat-free milk when you are thirsty. Soda and other sweet drinks contain a lot of sugar and are high in calories.

9 compare foods
Check out the **Food-A-Pedia** to look up and compare nutrition information for more than 8,000 foods.

10 make treats "treats," not everyday foods
Treats are great once in a while. Just don't make treat foods an everyday choice. Limit sweet treats to special occasions.

USDA
United States
Department of Agriculture
Center for Nutrition
Policy and Promotion

Go to www.ChooseMyPlate.gov for more information.

DG TipSheet No. 18
December 2011
USDA is an equal opportunity provider and employer.

Today's Date: _____

Making Healthy Eating Part of Your Total Lifestyle Evaluation

1=Strongly Disagree	2=Disagree	3=Neither Disagree or Agree		4=Agree		5=Strongly Agree

	1	2	3	4	5
1. The workshop covered useful information. Comments:	1	2	3	4	5
2. The workshop activities were helpful. Comments:	1	2	3	4	5
3. I will look at the Nutrition Facts Label when food shopping this week. Comments:	1	2	3	4	5
4. I plan to change my eating habits based on the information I learned today. Comments:	1	2	3	4	5
5. I plan to become more active based on the information learned today. Comments:	1	2	3	4	5
6. The instructor presented the information in a helpful way. Comments:	1	2	3	4	5
7. Overall, I found the workshop to be very helpful. Comments:	1	2	3	4	5

8. Please tell us which materials you found most useful.
Comments:

Workshop 6

Physical Activity Is Key to Living Well

Eat Healthy ● *Be Active*
Community Workshops

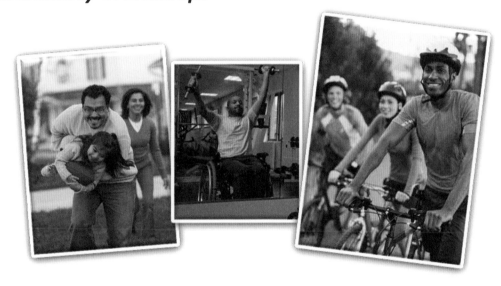

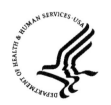

OFFICE OF
DISEASE
PREVENTION AND
HEALTH
PROMOTION

Instructor Guide

Before Workshop Begins

- Thoroughly read entire workshop and become familiar with the lesson plan.

- Choose an activity to do, and gather materials needed for the icebreaker and the chosen activity.

  - *Icebreaker*: Find Someone Who . . . handout for each participant, healthy prize items

  - *Activity 1*: Two soup cans or resistance bands of modest tension for each participant

  - *Activity 2* (Group Walk): Comfortable shoes to walk in

- *Note:* It would be a good idea to let participants know you will be doing some light exercising during this workshop and they may want to wear comfortable clothing and shoes.

- Photocopy handouts (one per participant):

  1. Be Active Your Way: A Fact Sheet for Adults (2 pages)
  2. Find Someone Who . . . (1 page)
  3. Muscle-Strengthening Exercises (6 pages)
  4. My Aerobic and Strengthening Activities Log (1 page)
  5. How Many Calories Does Physical Activity Use? (1 page)
  6. Workshop Evaluation (1 page)

Workshop Outline

The workshop should last ~1 hour, including activities.

- Icebreaker activity (5 minutes)—do this while people are coming into the workshop

- Introduction (5 minutes)

  - Explain the purpose of the workshop

  - Review the Learning Objectives

- **Objective 1:** Learn the benefits of physical activity and the specific recommendations for aerobic and strengthening activities (5–10 minutes)

  – Review handout: *Be Active Your Way: A Fact Sheet for Adults*

- **Objective 2:** Learn how to do strength-training activities (5 minutes)

  – Activity (10–15 minutes) Note: Choose ahead of time and gather supplies as needed

  – Review handout: *Muscle-Strengthening Exercises* (do activity with this)

- **Objective 3:** Learn how to develop and maintain a successful plan for physical activity. (5–10 minutes)

  – Review handout: *My Aerobic and Strengthening Activities Log*

- Wrap-up/Q&A (5 minutes)

  – Reminders of things to try at home:

    ▪ Work on increasing the amount of time you do physical activity each day

    ▪ Make a plan for physical activity (aerobic and strength training) and keep track of your progress

- Ask participants to complete the evaluation form (5 minutes)

Workshop Lesson Plan

Icebreaker Activity (5 minutes)

"Find Someone Who": This bingo-like game shows participants the many ways to stay active while letting them get to know one another. Pass out the game sheet and ask participants to walk around the room and talk to one another to learn which physical activities each likes to do. Participants then sign their names in the boxes for the activities they do. Depending on the size of the group, set a limit on how many boxes the same person can sign on a participant's game sheet (usually just two). Award a healthy prize (fruit, water bottle, jump rope, etc.) to the first person to get a complete row signed. To keep the game going, ask participants to try and complete two rows, a "T" pattern, or even the whole grid. It's helpful to have several prizes on hand to reward winners.

Supplies necessary: *Find Someone Who . . .* handout for each participant, healthy prize items.

Talking Points—Purpose of the Workshop (2–3 minutes)

- Today's workshop and handouts will give you tips on the amount of physical activity you need each day and ways to include physical activity as part of your daily routine.

- This workshop is based on the *Dietary Guidelines for Americans, 2010* and the *2008 Physical Activity Guidelines for Americans.* The Dietary Guidelines provide science-based advice for making food choices that promote good health and a healthy weight and help prevent disease. The Physical Activity Guidelines provide recommendations on the amount, types, and level of intensity of physical activity needed to achieve and maintain good health.

- The Dietary Guidelines provide these selected consumer messages. More information about the messages can be found at http://www.ChooseMyPlate.gov.

  - *Balancing Calories*
    - ✓ Enjoy your food, but eat less.
    - ✓ Avoid oversized portions.
  - *Foods to Increase*
    - ✓ Make half your plate fruits and vegetables.
    - ✓ Make at least half your grains whole grains.

       ✓ Switch to fat-free or low-fat (1%) milk.

– *Foods to Decrease*

       ✓ Compare sodium in foods like soup, bread, and frozen meals—and choose foods with lower numbers.

       ✓ Drink water instead of sugary drinks.

– Healthy eating and physical activity work hand in hand to help us live healthier lives. The Physical Activity Guidelines recommend that adults be physically active for at least 2 hours and 30 minutes each week—children need 60 minutes each day.

       ✓ You can stay physically active by doing activities such as walking, dancing, bicycling, or gardening and by reducing the amount of time you spend sitting.

Talking Points—Learning Objectives (2–3 minutes)

1. Learn the benefits of physical activity and the specific recommendations for aerobic and strengthening activities.

2. Learn how to do strength-training activities.

3. Learn how to develop and maintain a successful plan for physical activity.

Talking Points—Handout: Be Active Your Way Fact Sheet (5–10 minutes)

Getting Started

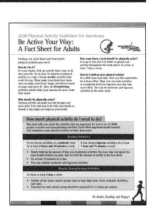

- Learn the benefits of physical activity.

  – Increase your chances for living longer.

  – Decrease risk of heart disease, type-2 diabetes, high blood pressure, high cholesterol, stroke, and some types of cancer (breast and colon).

  – Sleep better.

  – Fight depression.

  – Build strength.

  – Maintain a healthy weight.

  – Have fun!

How Much Physical Activity Do I Need?

Aerobic Activity

- Adults should get at least **2 hours and 30 minutes** each week of aerobic physical activity that requires <u>moderate</u> effort or **1 hour and 15 minutes** each week of aerobic physical activity that requires <u>vigorous</u> effort.

  - Adults need to do aerobic activity for at least 10 minutes at a time for health benefits.

  - Adults can do a combination of moderate and vigorous activities each week. In general, 1 minute of vigorous activity is equal to 2 minutes of moderate activity.

- Examples of <u>moderate aerobic activity</u> include walking briskly, biking slowly, canoeing, ballroom and line dancing, general gardening, doubles tennis, using a manual wheelchair, etc.

- Examples of <u>vigorous aerobic activity</u> include race walking, jogging, or running, biking fast, aerobic or fast dancing, heavy gardening (digging, hoeing), singles tennis, etc.

Muscle Strengthening Activity

- Adults also should do strengthening activities at least **2 days a week**.

- Examples of strengthening activities include pushups, situps, lifting weights, working with resistance bands, and heavy gardening.

  - Choose activities that work all the different parts of the body (legs, hips, back, chest, stomach, shoulders, and arms).

  - Exercises for each muscle group should be repeated 8 to 12 times per session.

Activity—Choose One Ahead of Time (10–15 minutes)

1. **Strengthening Exercises:** Using resistance bands (if you have them or can get them) or soup cans, demonstrate sample strengthening exercises from the National Institute on Aging. Select the exercises that work best given your physical space and type of chairs. Before working with participants, make sure that you have reviewed the exercises and tips. The arm raises, arm curls, and leg raises may be good ones for participants to try during the workshop.

   Supplies necessary: Two soup cans or resistance bands of modest tension for each participant

2. **Group Walk:** If you are unable to do a strengthening workout during the workshop, take participants on a 10–15 minute walk instead. Plan your route ahead of time and make sure it is safe and free of potholes and other things that could cause missteps or accidents.

Supplies necessary: Comfortable shoes to walk in

Note: It would be a good idea to let participants know you will be doing some light exercising during this workshop and they may want to wear comfortable clothing and shoes.

Talking Points—Handout: Muscle-Strengthening Exercises (5 minutes)

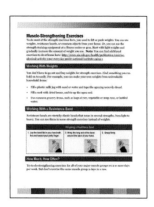

- Demonstrate that a repetition, or rep, is one complete movement of an exercise, and that a set is one group of reps—about 8–12 repetitions. Start out using light weights, such as 1- or 2-pound weights (a soup can usually weighs either 1 or 2 pounds). For those new to strength training, it's perfectly okay to start with no weights at all. Starting out with weights that are too heavy can cause injuries.

- Don't jerk or thrust weights into position. Use smooth, steady movements.

- Avoid locking your arm and leg joints in a tightly straightened position.

- Don't hold your breath. Breathe regularly.

- Muscle soreness lasting a few days and slight fatigue are normal after muscle-building exercises, at least at first.

- If you feel sick or have pain during or after exercise, you're doing too much.

- Over time, gradually increase the amount of weight used to build strength.

Refer participants to the *Muscle-Strengthening Exercises* handout and encourage them to try these exercises at home. More sample exercises can be found at http://www.nia.nih.gov/health/publication/exercise-physical-activity-your-everyday-guide-national-institute-aging-1.

Talking Points—Handout: My Aerobic and Strengthening Activities Log (5–10 minutes)

Getting Started

- Think about reasons why you have not been physically active. **Note:** You may want to have the participants share some of their reasons.

- Pick a physical activity that you like and one that fits into your life.

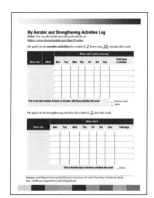

- Find the time that works best for you. Before work? After the kids go to bed? You decide!

- Be active with friends and family who can help you keep up with your physical activity plan.

- Consider using a pedometer to track your walking. Set goals to increase your number of steps every day or each week.

- There are health benefits of doing at least 10 minutes of physical activity at a time.

- Avoid sitting still—take advantage of all opportunities during the day to move!

  - Take the stairs instead of the elevator.

  - Park farther away in the parking lot.

  - Walk over to a coworker's desk instead of sending an e-mail.

Making Exercise Work for You

- Plan your activity for the week ahead of time.

  - Aim for at least 2 hours and 30 minutes of moderate physical activity each week.

    - It's best to spread aerobic activity out over at least 3 days a week.

  - Include strengthening activities 2 days a week to keep your muscles strong.

- Track your time and progress.

- Looking to add to your physical activity?

  - Work toward doubling your weekly activity time to 5 hours per week.

  - Replace some of your moderate-level aerobic activities with vigorous aerobic activities that make your heart beat even faster. In general, 15 minutes of vigorous activity provides the same benefits as 30 minutes of moderate activity.

– Vigorous activities include playing basketball, jogging/running, riding a bike faster or up hills, swimming laps, jumping rope, aerobic dance, etc.

– Add an extra day to your 2 days of strengthening activities.

• Mix it up: You can do all moderate activities, all vigorous activities, or some of each. Don't forget activities for stronger muscles.

• Avoid injury. You can do this by:

– Start slowly and build up to more activity.

– Choose activities that are appropriate for your level of fitness.

– Use the right safety gear and sports equipment.

– Choose a safe place to do your activity.

• **Sign Up:** Keep track of your physical activity (and nutrition goals!) by signing up for the Presidential Active Lifestyle Award (PALA+). You also can take small steps to improve your eating habits.

✓ If you are active for 30 minutes a day, 5 days a week for 6 out of 8 weeks, and choose one nutrition goal each week to work toward, you'll be awarded the PALA+ and receive Presidential recognition! (See http://www.presidentschallenge.org) See handout in Appendix for more information.

Talking Points—Wrap-up/Q&A (5 minutes)

Things to Try at Home

• Work on increasing the amount of time you do physical activity each day
• Make a plan for physical activity (aerobic and strength training) and keep track of your progress.

Complete Evaluation Form (5 minutes)

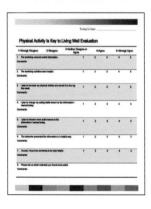

Workshop 6 ● Handouts

Be Active Your Way:
A Fact Sheet for Adults

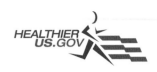

Finding out what kind and how much physical activity you need

How do I do it?
It's your choice. Pick an activity that's easy to fit into your life. Do at least 10 minutes of physical activity at a time. Choose **aerobic** activities that work for you. These make your heart beat faster and can make your heart, lungs, and blood vessels stronger and more fit. Also, do **strengthening** activities which make your muscles do more work than usual.

Why should I be physically active?
Physical activity can make you feel stronger and more alive. It is a fun way to be with your family or friends. It also helps you improve your health.

How many times a week should I be physically active?
It is up to you, but it is better to spread your activity throughout the week and to be active at least 3 days a week.

How do I build up more physical activity?
Do a little more each time. Once you feel comfortable, do it more often. Then you can trade activities at a moderate level for vigorous ones that take more effort. You can do moderate and vigorous activities in the same week.

How much physical activity do I need to do?

This chart tells you about the activities that are important for you to do. Do **both** aerobic activities and strengthening activities. Each offers important health benefits. And remember, some physical activity is better than none!

Aerobic Activities

If you choose activities at a **moderate** level, do at least **2 hours and 30 minutes** a week.	If you choose **vigorous** activities, do at least **1 hour and 15 minutes** a week.

- Slowly build up the amount of time you do physical activities. The more time you spend, the more health benefits you gain. Aim for twice the amount of activity in the box above.
- Do at least 10 minutes at a time.
- You can combine moderate and vigorous activities.

Muscle Strengthening Activities

Do these at least **2 days** a week.

- Include all the major muscle groups such as legs, hips, back, chest, stomach, shoulders, and arms.
- Exercises for each muscle group should be repeated 8 to 12 times per session.

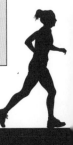

Be Active, Healthy, and Happy!

How can I tell an activity at a moderate level from a vigorous one?

Vigorous activities take more effort than moderate ones. Here are just a few moderate and vigorous aerobic physical activities. Do these for **10 minutes or more** at a time.

Moderate Activities	Vigorous Activities
(I can talk while I do them, but I can't sing.)	(I can only say a few words without stopping to catch my breath.)
• Ballroom and line dancing	• Aerobic dance
• Biking on level ground or with few hills	• Biking faster than 10 miles per hour
• Canoeing	• Fast dancing
• General gardening (raking, trimming shrubs)	• Heavy gardening (digging, hoeing)
• Sports where you catch and throw (baseball, softball, volleyball)	• Hiking uphill
• Tennis (doubles)	• Jumping rope
• Using your manual wheelchair	• Martial arts (such as karate)
• Using hand cyclers—also called ergometers	• Race walking, jogging, or running
• Walking briskly	• Sports with a lot of running (basketball, hockey, soccer)
• Water aerobics	• Swimming fast or swimming laps
	• Tennis (singles)

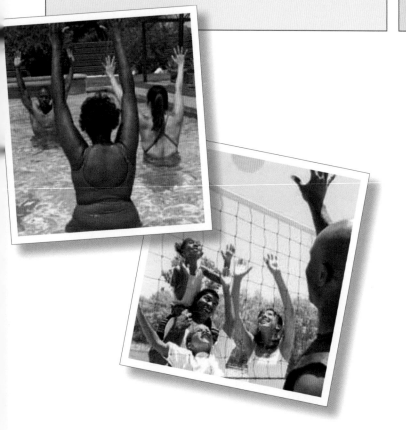

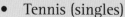

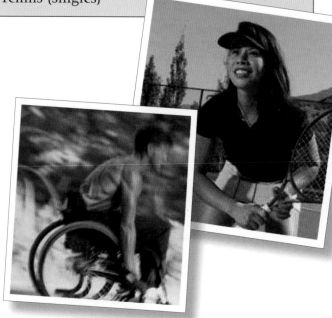

For more information, visit www.healthfinder.gov/getactive

Be active **your way** by choosing activities you enjoy!

ODPHP Publication No. U0038

October 2008

Find Someone Who . . .

How Do You Stay Active?

Went for a bike ride this week	Likes to swim	Has run in a race before	Goes for a brisk walk on most days
Likes to play tennis	Has jumped rope as an adult	Plays on a sports team	Engaged in aerobic exercise three times last week
Feels good after exercising	Has used a pedometer before	Enjoys canoeing or kayaking	Works in the garden
Prefers to exercise in the morning	Has weights at home	Has tried yoga or Pilates	Prefers to exercise in the evening

Muscle-Strengthening Exercises

To do most of the strength exercises here, you need to lift or push weights. You can use weights, resistance bands, or common objects from your home. Or, you can use the strength-training equipment at a fitness center or gym. Start with light weights and gradually increase the amount of weight you use. **Note:** You can find additional exercises to do at home here: http://www.nia.nih.gov/health/publication/exercise-physical-activity-your-everyday-guide-national-institute-aging-1

Working With Weights

You don't have to go out and buy weights for strength exercises. Find something you can hold on to easily. For example, you can make your own weights from unbreakable household items:

- Fill a plastic milk jug with sand or water and tape the opening securely closed.

- Fill a sock with dried beans, and tie up the open end.

- Use common grocery items, such as bags of rice, vegetable or soup cans, or bottled water.

Working With a Resistance Band

Resistance bands are stretchy elastic bands that come in several strengths, from light to heavy. You can use them in some strength exercises instead of weights.

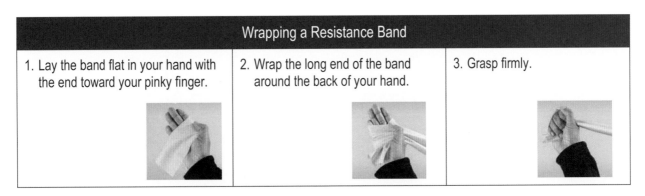

Wrapping a Resistance Band		
1. Lay the band flat in your hand with the end toward your pinky finger.	2. Wrap the long end of the band around the back of your hand.	3. Grasp firmly.

How Much, How Often?

Try to do strengthening exercises for all of your major muscle groups on 2 or more days per week. But don't exercise the same muscle group 2 days in a row.

- If you have not done strength training before, you might need to start out using 1- or 2-pound weights (or no weights at all). Your body needs to get used to strength exercises. Starting out with weights that are too heavy can cause injuries.

- It should feel somewhere between hard and very hard for you to lift the weight. It shouldn't feel very, very hard. If you can't lift a weight 8 times in a row, it's too heavy for you. Reduce the amount of weight.

- Take 3 seconds to lift or push a weight into place, hold the position for 1 second, and take another 3 seconds to return to your starting position. Don't let the weight drop; returning it slowly is very important. This is one complete movement of an exercise, or a repetition.

- Start by lifting 8 times, working up to 8–12 repetitions for each exercise. If you can't do that many at first, do as many as you can. You may be able to build up to this goal over time.

- When you can do two sets of 8–12 repetitions easily, increase the amount of weight at the next session. Keep repeating until you can reach your goal, and then maintain that level as long as you can.

Safety

- Talk with your doctor if you are unsure about doing a particular exercise. For example, if you've had hip or back surgery, talk about which exercises might be best for you.

- Don't hold your breath during strength exercises. Holding your breath while straining can cause changes in blood pressure. This is especially true for people with heart disease. Breathe regularly.

- Proper form and safety go hand-in-hand. For some exercises, you may want to start by alternating arms and work your way up to using both arms at the same time. If it is difficult for you to hold hand weights, try using wrist weights.

- To prevent injury, don't jerk or thrust weights into position. Use smooth, steady movements.

- Avoid "locking" your arm and leg joints in a tightly straightened position. To straighten your knees, tighten your thigh muscles. This will lift your kneecaps and protect them.

- For many of the sample exercises in this guide, you will need to use a chair. Choose a sturdy chair that is stable enough to support your weight when seated or when holding on during the exercise.

- Muscle soreness lasting a few days and slight fatigue are normal after muscle-building exercises, at least at first. After doing these exercises for a few weeks, you will probably not be sore after your workout.

Overhead Arm Raise

This exercise will strengthen your shoulders and arms. It should make swimming and other activities such as lifting and carrying heavy items easier.

1. You can do this exercise while standing or sitting in a sturdy, armless chair. Hold weight with palm facing upward.
2. Keep your feet flat on the floor, shoulder-width apart.
3. Hold weights at your sides at shoulder height with palms facing forward. Breathe in slowly.
4. Slowly breathe out as you raise both arms up over your head, keeping your elbows slightly bent.
5. Hold the position for 1 second.
6. Breathe in as you slowly lower your arms.
7. Repeat 8–12 times.
8. Rest; then repeat 8–12 more times.
9. As you progress, use a heavier weight and alternate arms until you can lift the weight comfortably with both arms.

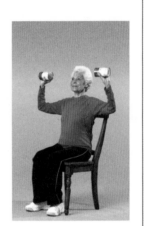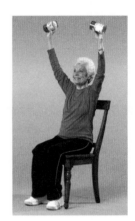

Front Arm Raise

This exercise will strengthen your shoulders and make lifting groceries easier.

1. Stand with your feet shoulder-width apart. Keep your feet flat on the floor during the exercise.
2. Hold weights straight down at your sides, with palms facing backward.
3. Keeping them straight, breathe out as you raise both arms in front of you to shoulder height.
4. Hold the position for 1 second.
5. Breathe in as you slowly lower your arms.
6. Repeat 8–12 times.
7. Rest; then repeat 8–12 more times.
8. As you progress, use a heavier weight and alternate arms until you can lift the weight comfortably with both arms.

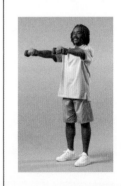

Side Arm Raise

This exercise for your shoulders can help you put things up on a shelf or take them down more easily.

1. You can do this exercise while standing or sitting in a sturdy, armless chair.
2. Keep your feet flat on the floor, shoulder-width apart.
3. Hold hand weights straight down at your sides with palms facing inward. Breathe in slowly.
4. Slowly breathe out as you raise both arms to the side, to shoulder height.
5. Hold the position for 1 second.
6. Breathe in as you slowly lower your arms.
7. Repeat 8–12 times.
8. Rest; then repeat 8–12 more times.
9. As you progress, use a heavier weight and alternate arms until you can lift the weight comfortably with both arms.

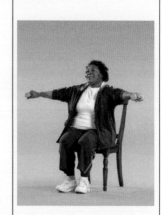

Arm Curl

After a few weeks of doing this exercise for your upper arm muscles, lifting that gallon of milk will be much easier.

1. Stand with your feet shoulder-width apart.
2. Hold weights straight down at your sides, palms facing forward. Breathe in slowly.
3. Breathe out as you slowly bend your elbows and lift weights toward chest. Keep elbows at your sides.
4. Hold the position for 1 second.
5. Breathe in as you slowly lower your arms.
6. Repeat 8–12 times.
7. Rest; then repeat 8–12 more times.
8. As you progress, use a heavier weight and alternate arms until you can lift the weight comfortably with both arms.

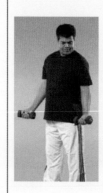 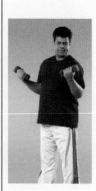

Arm Curl With Resistance Band

This variation of the Arm Curl uses a resistance band instead of weights.

1. Sit in a sturdy, armless chair with your feet flat on the floor, shoulder-width apart.
2. Place the center of the resistance band under both feet. Hold each end of the band with palms facing inward. Keep elbows at your sides. Breathe in slowly.
3. Keep wrists straight and slowly breathe out as you bend your elbows and bring your hands toward your shoulders.
4. Hold the position for 1 second.
5. Breathe in as you slowly lower your arms.
6. Repeat 8–12 times.
7. Rest; then repeat 8–12 more times.
8. As you progress, use a heavier strength band.

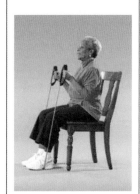

Back Leg Raise

This exercise strengthens your buttocks and lower back. For an added challenge, you can modify the exercise to improve your balance.

1. Stand behind a sturdy chair, holding on for balance. Breathe in slowly.
2. Breathe out and slowly lift one leg straight back without bending your knee or pointing your toes. Try not to lean forward. The leg you are standing on should be slightly bent.
3. Hold position for 1 second.
4. Breathe in as you slowly lower your leg.
5. Repeat 8–12 times.
6. Repeat 8–12 times with other leg.
7. Repeat 8–12 more times with each leg.
8. As you progress, you may want to add ankle weights.

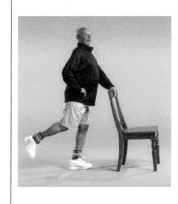

Side Leg Raise

This exercise strengthens hips, thighs, and buttocks. For an added challenge, you can modify the exercise to improve your balance.

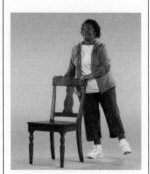

1. Stand behind a sturdy chair with feet slightly apart, holding on for balance. Breathe in slowly.
2. Breathe out and slowly lift one leg out to the side. Keep your back straight and your toes facing forward. The leg you are standing on should be slightly bent.
3. Hold position for 1 second.
4. Breathe in as you slowly lower your leg.
5. Repeat 8–12 times.
6. Repeat 8–12 times with other leg.
7. Repeat 8–12 more times with each leg.
8. As you progress, you may want to add ankle weights.

My Aerobic and Strengthening Activities Log

Note: You can also track your physical activity at:
https://www.choosemyplate.gov/SuperTracker

My goal is to do **aerobic activities** for a total of <u>2</u> hours and <u>30</u> minutes this week.

What I did	Effort	When I did it and for how long							Total hours or minutes
		Mon	Tue	Wed	Thu	Fri	Sat	Sun	

This is the total number of hours or minutes I did these activities this week: ___ *hours and* ___ *min*

My goal is to do strengthening activities for a total of <u>2</u> days this week.

What I did	When I did it							Total days
	Mon	Tue	Wed	Thu	Fri	Sat	Sun	

This is the total days I did these activities this week: ___ *days*

Source: *2008 Physical Activity Guidelines for Americans,* Be Active Your Way: A Guide for Adults.
http://health.gov/paguidelines/pdf/adultguide.pdf

How Many Calories Does Physical Activity Use?

The number of calories varies depending on many factors including weight, age, and environmental conditions. This chart provides an estimate for the number of calories males and females may burn doing various activities for 10 minutes at a time.

Physical Activity Level	Approximate Calories Burned in 10 minutes	
	Men (175–250 lbs)	Women (140–200 lbs)
Moderate Physical Activity		
Ballroom and line dancing	50–80	40–60
Bicycling on level ground or with a few hills		
General gardening (raking, trimming shrubs)		
Sports where you catch and throw (baseball, softball, volleyball)		
Tennis (doubles)		
Using your manual wheelchair		
Walking briskly		
Water aerobics		
Vigorous Physical Activity		
Aerobic dance or fast dance	120–150	100–120
Biking faster than 10 miles per hour		
Heavy gardening (digging, hoeing)		
Hiking uphill		
Jumping rope		
Martial arts (such as karate)		
Race walking, jogging, running		
Sports with a lot of running (basketball, hockey, soccer, singles tennis)		
Swimming fast or swimming laps		

Source: Adapted from Move Virginia, Calories Burned During Physical Activities.
http://www.move.va.gov/download/NewHandouts/PhysicalActivity/
P03_CaloriesBurnedDuringPhysicalActivities.pdf

Today's Date: _____

Physical Activity Is Key to Living Well Evaluation

1=Strongly Disagree	2=Disagree	3=Neither Disagree or Agree	4=Agree	5=Strongly Agree

	1	2	3	4	5
1. The workshop covered useful information. Comments:	1	2	3	4	5
2. The workshop activities were helpful. Comments:	1	2	3	4	5
3. I plan to increase my physical activity and record it on the log this week. Comments:	1	2	3	4	5
4. I plan to change my eating habits based on the information I learned today. Comments:	1	2	3	4	5
5. I plan to become more active based on the information I learned today. Comments:	1	2	3	4	5
6. The instructor presented the information in a helpful way. Comments:	1	2	3	4	5
7. Overall, I found the workshop to be very helpful. Comments:	1	2	3	4	5

8. Please tell us which materials you found most useful.

Comments:

Appendix ● Additional Resources

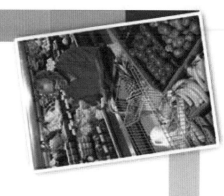

[Insert your
Organization
Logo here.
Size .8x.8" max]

Certificate of Completion

presented to

Insert Name of Recipient

For participating in the

Eat Healthy • Be Active

Community Workshops

*based on the Dietary Guidelines for Americans 2010 and
2008 Physical Activity Guidelines for Americans*

[Insert MM/DD/YEAR]

_____

[Insert Name, Title]

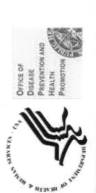

Office of
Disease
Prevention and
Health
Promotion

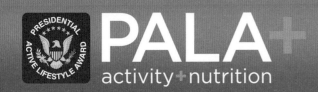

Be active. Have fun.

Presidential Active Lifestyle Award: Activity + Nutrition (PALA+)

PALA+ promotes physical activity AND good nutrition, because it takes both to lead a healthy lifestyle. Sign up for the six-week program to help you maintain or improve your health. Anyone age 6 and older can earn their PALA+ today – sign up at **www.presidentschallenge.org** or use the log on the reverse side.

PHYSICAL ACTIVITY A healthy life is an active life. Youth (6-17 years old) need to be active at least 60 minutes a day (or 11,000 steps for girls and 13,000 steps for boys). Adults (18 and older), 30 minutes (or 8500 steps). So, take a walk with friends, bike ride after dinner, garden, or play a game of basketball at the park. Get your heart pumping and your muscles moving. When you've logged six weeks of physical activity, congratulations. You've started a regular routine for a more active lifestyle.

GOOD NUTRITION
Start eating healthy. It's easier than you think! Take it one step at a time. Commit to one new healthy eating goal this week, and circle it on your weekly PALA+ log. The following week add a different goal – but make sure you continue to maintain your healthy eating goal(s) from the week(s) before. Focus on your healthy eating goals every week and remember, the more often you incorporate them into your lifestyle, the better you will feel. When you've achieved six different healthy eating goals, congratulations. You've started a routine for a healthier lifestyle.

Tips for Healthy Eating:

Make half your plate fruit and vegetables.

Keep it simple by filling half your plate with fruits and vegetables at meal time. The more colorful you make your plate; the more likely you are to get the vitamins, minerals, and fiber your body needs to be healthy. Remember that all forms count – fresh, frozen, canned (fruit in water or 100% juice), dried, or 100% juice.

Make half the grains you eat whole grains.

An easy way to eat more whole grains is to switch from a refined grain food to a whole-grain food. For example, eat whole-wheat bread instead of white bread, brown rice instead of white rice, and low-fat popcorn instead of snack chips. Read the ingredients list and choose products that list a whole-grain ingredient first. Look for things like: "whole wheat," "brown rice," "bulgur," "buckwheat," "oatmeal," "rolled oats," "quinoa," or "wild rice."

Choose fat-free or low-fat (1%) milk, yogurt, or cheese.

To help build your bones and keep them strong, dairy products should be a key part of your diet because they provide calcium, vitamin D, and many other nutrients your bones need.

Drink water instead of sugary drinks.

Regular soda and other sweet drinks such as fruit drinks and energy drinks are high in calories because they have a lot of added sugar. Instead, reach for a tall glass of water. Try adding a slice of lemon, lime or watermelon or a splash of 100% juice to your glass of water if you want some flavor.

Choose lean sources of protein.

Meat, poultry, seafood, dry beans or peas, eggs, nuts, and seeds are considered part of the protein foods group. Select leaner cuts of ground beef (label says 90% lean or higher), turkey breast, or chicken breast. Grill, roast, poach, or boil meat, poultry, or seafood instead of frying. Include beans or peas in main dishes such as chili, stews, casseroles, salads, tacos, enchiladas, and burritos.

Compare sodium in foods like soup and frozen meals and choose foods with less sodium.

Read the Nutrition Facts label to compare sodium in foods like soup, bread, canned vegetables, and frozen meals – and choose the foods with lower amounts. Look for "low sodium," "reduced sodium," and "no salt added" on food packages.

Eat some seafood.

Seafood includes fish (such as salmon, tuna, and trout) and shellfish (such as crab, mussels, and oysters). Seafood has protein, minerals, and omega-3 fatty acids (heart healthy fat). Adults should try to eat at least 8 ounces a week of a variety of seafood. Children can eat smaller amounts of seafood too.

Pay attention to portion size.
Check to see what the recommended portion sizes of

foods you eat look like in the bowls, plates, and glasses you use at home. For example – check 3/4 cup cereal, 3 ounces cooked chicken, 1 cup milk, 1/2 cup of juice. When dining out avoid "supersizing" your meal or buying "combo" meal deals that often include large size menu items. Choose small size items instead or ask for a "take home" bag and wrap up half of your meal to take home before you even start to eat.

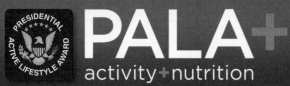

PALA+
activity+nutrition

PRESIDENTIAL ACTIVE LIFESTYLE AWARD

PRESIDENT'S CHALLENGE PROGRAM

PRESIDENT'S COUNCIL ON FITNESS, SPORTS & NUTRITION

www.presidentschallenge.org

Participant Name _____ Age _____ Date Started _____

Group ID (if applicable) _____ Date Completed _____

Week 1

Day	Physical Activities	# of Minutes or Pedometer Steps
Mon		
Tues		
Wed		
Thurs		
Fri		
Sat		
Sun		

Healthy Eating—Select a goal for this week.

Week 2

Day	Physical Activities	# of Minutes or Pedometer Steps
Mon		
Tues		
Wed		
Thurs		
Fri		
Sat		
Sun		

Healthy Eating—Circle and continue with last week's goal, and add a new goal.

Week 3

Day	Physical Activities	# of Minutes or Pedometer Steps
Mon		
Tues		
Wed		
Thurs		
Fri		
Sat		
Sun		

Healthy Eating—Circle and continue with previous goals, and add a new goal.

Week 4

Day	Physical Activities	# of Minutes or Pedometer Steps
Mon		
Tues		
Wed		
Thurs		
Fri		
Sat		
Sun		

Healthy Eating—Circle and continue with previous goals, and add a new goal.

Week 5

Day	Physical Activities	# of Minutes or Pedometer Steps
Mon		
Tues		
Wed		
Thurs		
Fri		
Sat		
Sun		

Healthy Eating—Circle and continue with previous goals, and add a new goal.

Week 6

Day	Physical Activities	# of Minutes or Pedometer Steps
Mon		
Tues		
Wed		
Thurs		
Fri		
Sat		
Sun		

Healthy Eating—Circle and continue with previous goals, and add a new goal.

Healthy Eating Goals

- I made half my plate fruits and vegetables
- At least half of the grains that I ate were whole grains
- I chose fat-free or low fat (1%) milk, yogurt, or cheese
- I drank water instead of sugary drinks
- I chose lean sources of protein
- I compared sodium in foods like soup and frozen meals and chose foods with less sodium
- I ate seafood
- I ate smaller portions

INSTRUCTIONS: Online: Create an online account at www.presidentschallenge.org. Participate as an individual or join a group (ID at the top of page if applicable). Once you achieve PALA, you're eligible to receive a certificate! **Paper:** Use this hard copy log to track your progress. Once completed, report your accomplishment and receive your certificate at www.presidentschallenge.org! Or, if part of a group, make sure to return it to your group administrator to get recognized.

CLEAN

- Washing hands with soap and warm water before and after handling raw food is the best way to reduce the spread of germs and prevent food poisoning.

- Thoroughly wash utensils, cutting boards, and countertops with soap and hot water. Rinse. They may be sanitized by applying a solution of 1 tablespoon of unscented, liquid chlorine bleach per gallon of water. Air-dry.

- Wash fruits and vegetables thoroughly under running water just before eating, cutting, or cooking. Washing fruits and vegetables with soap or detergent or using commercial produce washes is not recommended.

1 in 6 Americans will get sick from food poisoning this year. 3,000 Americans will die. Keep your family food safer.

Raw milk and products made from raw milk (including certain cheeses, ice cream, and yogurt) are foods that can pose severe health risks. Raw milk and products made from raw milk can carry harmful bacteria and other germs that can make you very sick or kill you. At the grocery store, look for milk and milk products that are labeled "pasteurized" (which means the milk has been heated briefly to kill disease-causing germs). If you do not see the word "pasteurized" on the product label, the product may contain raw milk. Pasteurized milk and milk products are safer than raw milk and products made from raw milk.

SEPARATE

- Keep raw meat, poultry, eggs, and seafood and their juices away from ready-to-eat food.

- Separate raw meat, poultry, and seafood from produce in your shopping cart. Place food in plastic bags to prevent their juices, which may contain harmful bacteria, from dripping onto other food.

- At home, put raw meat, poultry, and seafood in containers, on plates, or in sealed plastic bags in the refrigerator to prevent their juices from dripping onto other food.

- Use a separate cutting board for raw meat, poultry, and seafood.

- Sauce that is used to marinate raw meat, poultry, or seafood should not be used on cooked food, unless the sauce is boiled first.

- Never place cooked food back on the same plate that previously held raw food unless the plate has first been washed in hot, soapy water.

COOK

- Color and texture are unreliable indicators of safety. Using a food thermometer is the only way to ensure the safety of meat, poultry, seafood, and egg products. These foods must be cooked to a safe minimum internal temperature to destroy any harmful bacteria.

- The food thermometer should be placed in the thickest part of the food, away from bone, fat, or gristle.

Safe Minimum Internal Temperatures
As measured with a food thermometer

Beef, pork, veal and lamb (roast, steaks and chops)	145 °F with a 3-minute "rest time" after removal from the heat source.
Ground Meats	160 °F
Poultry (whole, parts or ground)	165 °F
Eggs and egg dishes	160 °F Cook eggs until both the yolk and the white are firm. Scrambled eggs should not be runny.
Leftovers	165 °F
Fin Fish	145 °F

Safe Cooking Guidelines

Shrimp, Lobster, Crabs	Flesh pearly and opaque
Clams, Oysters and Mussels	Shells open during cooking
Scallops	Milky white, opaque and firm

CHILL

※ The temperature in a refrigerator should be 40 °F or below, and the freezer 0 °F or below.

※ Perishable food should be thawed in the refrigerator, in the microwave, or in cold water. They should never be thawed on the counter or in hot water. Do not leave food at room temperature for more than two hours (one hour when the temperature is above 90 °F).

※ Meat and poultry defrosted in the refrigerator may be refrozen before or after cooking. If thawed in the microwave or cold water, cook before refreezing.

※ Divide large pots of food, like soup or stew, into shallow containers. Cut cooked meat or poultry into smaller portions or slices. Place in shallow containers, cover, and refrigerate.

※ Only buy eggs from a refrigerator or refrigerated case. Store eggs in the refrigerator in their original carton and use within 3-5 weeks.

※ When selecting pre-cut produce choose only those items that are refrigerated or surrounded by ice and keep refrigerated at home to maintain both quality and safety.

KEEP YOUR FAMILY SAFER FROM FOOD POISONING

Check your steps at FoodSafety.gov

Additional Resources

There are many more resources and materials to help you promote healthy eating and physical activity in your community. The following sections include the titles of materials available from the U.S. Department of Agriculture (USDA), additional helpful recipes and menus, more information about the Dietary Guidelines and Physical Activity Guidelines, and a list of Federal resources related to nutrition and physical activity.

Helpful Materials

The USDA has produced many helpful materials—"Let's Eat for the Health of It" (http://www.choosemyplate.gov/food-groups/downloads/MyPlate/DG2010Brochure.pdf) offers a wide range of practical tips and appealing photos that reflect key recommendations from the guidelines.

The USDA's 10 Tips Nutrition Education Series (http://www.choosemyplate.gov/healthy-eating-tips/ten-tips.html) provides consumers and professionals with high-quality, easy-to-follow tips in a convenient, printable format. These are perfect for posting on a refrigerator. A different *Ten Tips* handout has been included in each of the six workshops. There are many other helpful tip sheets in the series, with more being added:

- Choose MyPlate: http://www.choosemyplate.gov/food-groups/downloads/TenTips/DGTipsheet1ChooseMyPlate.pdf

- Add More Vegetables to Your Day: http://www.choosemyplate.gov/food-groups/downloads/TenTips/DGTipsheet2AddMoreVegetables.pdf

- Focus on Fruits: http://www.choosemyplate.gov/food-groups/downloads/TenTips/DGTipsheet3FocusOnFruits.pdf

- Make Half Your Grains Whole: http://www.choosemyplate.gov/food-groups/downloads/TenTips/DGTipsheet4MakeHalfYourGrainsWhole.pdf

- Got Your Dairy Today?: http://www.choosemyplate.gov/food-groups/downloads/TenTips/DGTipsheet5GotYourDairyToday.pdf

- Build a Healthy Meal: http://www.choosemyplate.gov/food-groups/downloads/TenTips/DGTipsheet7BuildAHealthyMeal.pdf

- Healthy Eating for Vegetarians: http://www.choosemyplate.gov/food-groups/downloads/TenTips/DGTipsheet8HealthyEatingForVegetarians.pdf

- Smart Shopping for Veggies and Fruits: http://www.choosemyplate.gov/food-groups/downloads/TenTips/DGTipsheet9SmartShopping.pdf

- Liven up Your Meals With Vegetables and Fruits: http://www.choosemyplate.gov/foodgroups/downloads/TenTips/DGTipsheet10LivenUpYourMeals.pdf

- Kid-Friendly Veggies and Fruits: http://www.choosemyplate.gov/food-groups/downloads/TenTips/DGTipsheet11KidFriendlyVeggiesAndFruits.pdf

- Be a Healthy Role Model for Children: http://www.choosemyplate.gov/food-groups/downloads/TenTips/DGTipsheet12BeAHealthyRoleModel.pdf

- Cut Back on Your Kid's Sweet Treats: http://www.choosemyplate.gov/food-groups/downloads/TenTips/DGTipsheet13CutBackOnSweetTreats.pdf

- Salt and Sodium: http://www.choosemyplate.gov/food-groups/downloads/TenTips/DGTipsheet14SaltAndSodium.pdf

- Eat Seafood Twice a Week: http://www.choosemyplate.gov/food-groups/downloads/TenTips/DGTipsheet15EatSeafood.pdf

- Eating Better on a Budget: http://www.choosemyplate.gov/food-groups/downloads/TenTips/DGTipsheet16EatingBetterOnABudget.pdf

- Use SuperTracker Your Way: http://www.choosemyplate.gov/food-groups/downloads/TenTips/DGTipsheet17SuperTracker.pdf

- Enjoy Your Food, But Eat Less: http://www.choosemyplate.gov/food-groups/downloads/TenTips/DGTipsheet18EnjoyYourFood.pdf

Helpful Resources

The following Federal Government resources provide reliable, science-based information on nutrition and physical activity, as well as an evolving array of tools to facilitate Americans' adoption of healthy choices.

Federal Guidelines

- *Dietary Guidelines for Americans, 2010:*
  http://www.health.gov/dietaryguidelines

- *2008 Physical Activity Guidelines for Americans:*
  http://www.health.gov/paguidelines

Nutrition

- U.S. Department of Health and Human Services
  - Health.gov: http://health.gov
  - Healthfinder.gov: http://www.healthfinder.gov
  - Healthy People: http://www.healthypeople.gov
  - Office of Disease Prevention and Health Promotion: http://odphp.hhs.gov
  - Office of the Surgeon General—Childhood Overweight and Obesity Prevention Initiative: http://www.surgeongeneral.gov/obesityprevention/index.html
  - Centers for Disease Control and Prevention: http://www.cdc.gov
  - Food and Drug Administration: http://www.fda.gov
  - National Institutes of Health—***We Can!*** (Ways to Enhance Children's Activity and Nutrition): http://www.nhlbi.nih.gov/health/public/heart/obesity/wecan/
  - *Let's Move!*: http://www.letsmove.gov (Nutrition and physical activity information)
- U.S. Department of Agriculture
  - ChooseMyPlate: http://www.choosemyplate.gov/
  - Nutrition.gov: http://www.nutrition.gov
  - Center for Nutrition Policy and Promotion: http://www.cnpp.usda.gov
  - Food and Nutrition Service: http://www.fns.usda.gov
  - Team Nutrition: http://www.fns.usda.gov/tn
  - Food and Nutrition Information Center: http://fnic.nal.usda.gov
  - National Institute of Food and Agriculture: http://www.nifa.usda.gov
- Recipes and Menus
  - http://www.choosemyplate.gov/healthy-eating-tips/sample-menus-recipes.html
  - http://healthymeals.nal.usda.gov/schoolmeals/Recipes/recipefinder.php
  - http://www.nhlbi.nih.gov/health/public/heart/other/ktb_recipebk/famrec.htm
- Food Safety
  - Food Safety Basics: http://www.foodsafety.gov/keep/basics/

- – Educational Materials and Campaigns: http://www.fsis.usda.gov/Food_Safety_Education/Available_Downloads/index.asp
- – Safe Food Handling: http://www.fsis.usda.gov/Fact_Sheets/7_Steps_Community_Meals/index.asp
- – CDC Vital Signs, Making Food Safer to Eat: http://www.cdc.gov/vitalsigns/FoodSafety/index.html

- Nutrition Facts Label

  - – http://www.fda.gov/Food/ResourcesForYou/Consumers/NFLPM/default.htm

- Portion Sizes

  - – Portion Distortion Quiz from NHLBI: http://hp2010.nhlbihin.net/portion/

  - – How Many Fruits and Vegetables Do You Need?: http://www.fruitsandveggiesmatter.gov/

  - – Just Enough for You: http://www.win.niddk.nih.gov/publications/just_enough.htm

- Body Mass Index (BMI)

  - – http://www.cdc.gov/healthyweight/assessing/bmi/

  - – http://www.nhlbisupport.com/bmi/

Physical Activity

- President's Council on Fitness, Sports, and Nutrition: http://www.presidentschallenge.org

  http://www.fitness.gov

- Centers for Disease Control and Prevention: http://www.cdc.gov

  - – Division of Adolescent and School Health: http://www.cdc.gov/HealthyYouth/physicalactivity

  - – Division of Nutrition, Physical Activity, and Obesity: http://www.cdc.gov/nccdphp/dnpa/physical/index.htm

  - – Healthier Worksite Initiative: http://www.cdc.gov/nccdphp/dnpa/hwi/index.htm

- National Physical Activity Plan: http://www.physicalactivityplan.org/

- Sample Exercises and Information on Physical Activity
  http://www.nia.nih.gov/health/publication/exercise-physical-activity-your-everyday-guide-national-institute-aging-1

Answering Questions About the Guidelines

The following information has been extracted from frequently asked questions for each set of guidelines (posted on their respective Web sites). A complete set of questions and answers can be found at http://www.health.gov/dietaryguidelines/faq.asp and http://www.health.gov/paguidelines/faqs.aspx.

Dietary Guidelines for Americans, 2010

What are the Dietary Guidelines?

The Dietary Guidelines provide advice for making food choices that promote good health and a healthy weight and help prevent disease for healthy Americans aged 2 years and older. The advice is based on a rigorous review of the scientific evidence through a transparent, unbiased process. The Dietary Guidelines are congressionally mandated under the 1990 National Nutrition Monitoring and Related Research Act (Public Law 101-445, Section 301 [7 U.S.C. 5341], Title III). The guidelines are released by the Secretaries of the USDA and Health and Human Services (HHS) every 5 years.

Why are the Dietary Guidelines important?

They form the basis of Federal nutrition policy, education, outreach, and food assistance programs used by consumers, industry, nutrition educators, and health professionals. All Federal dietary guidance for the public is required to be consistent with the Dietary Guidelines. The guidelines provide the scientific basis for the Government to speak in a consistent and uniform manner. They are used in the development of materials, messages, tools, and programs to communicate healthy eating and physical activity to the public.

2008 Physical Activity Guidelines for Americans

Why should people be more physically active?

HHS published physical activity guidelines for the first time because being physically active is one of the most important steps that Americans of all ages can take to improve their health. The *2008 Physical Activity Guidelines for Americans* provide science-based guidance to help Americans aged 6 years and older improve their health through appropriate physical activity. These guidelines are necessary because of the importance of physical activity to the health of Americans, whose current inactivity puts them at unnecessary risk. Unfortunately, the latest data show that inactivity among American adults and youth remains relatively high and little progress has been made in increasing the level of physical activity in the population.

What are the Physical Activity Guidelines for adults?

Adults should do a minimum of 2 hours and 30 minutes of moderate-intensity aerobic activity a week by doing activities like brisk walking, ballroom dancing, or general gardening. Or adults can choose 1 hour and 15 minutes (75 minutes) a week of vigorous-intensity aerobic physical activity by doing activities like jogging, aerobic dancing, and jumping rope. Adults also may choose combinations of moderate- and vigorous-intensity aerobic activity. In general, 1 minute of vigorous activity is equal to 2 minutes of moderate activity.

Aerobic activity should be performed in episodes of at least 10 minutes, preferably spread throughout the week. For additional and more extensive health benefits, adults should increase their aerobic physical activity to 5 hours (300 minutes) a week of moderate-intensity, 2 hours and 30 minutes a week of vigorous-intensity, or an equivalent combination of moderate- and vigorous-intensity aerobic physical activity. Additional health benefits are gained by engaging in physical activity beyond this amount. Adults also should do muscle-strengthening activities on 2 or more days a week to achieve the unique benefits of strengthening activities.

What are the Physical Activity Guidelines for children and adolescents?

Children and adolescents aged 6–17 years should accumulate 1 hour or more of physical activity daily. The 1 hour of activity should be mostly aerobic but also should include muscle-strengthening and bone-strengthening activities. Youth should include vigorous-intensity activity in this 1 hour on at least 3 days a week. They also should do muscle-strengthening activities on at least 3 days and bone-strengthening activities on at least 3 days a week. It is important to encourage young people to participate in physical activities that are appropriate for their age, enjoyable, and offer variety. The guidelines list a number of examples of each type of activity for children and adolescents.

Answering Questions About MyPlate

What was the reasoning for developing the new MyPlate icon?

MyPlate was developed as an effort to promote healthy eating to consumers. The MyPlate icon is easy to understand and it helps promote messages based on the *Dietary Guidelines for Americans, 2010*. The new MyPlate icon builds on a familiar image—a plate—and is accompanied by messages to encourage consumers to make healthy choices.

Physical activity is not illustrated on the MyPlate icon. What is the rationale for the change?

To simplify the image, the MyPlate icon includes only the five food groups to help remind consumers to eat healthfully. It does not include all of the messages of the Dietary Guidelines. Although not depicted in this icon, physical activity is still very important for an overall healthy lifestyle. Balancing healthy eating with regular physical activity is essential, and the principles found in the *2008 Physical Activity Guidelines for Americans* "Be Active Your Way" handout will be emphasized throughout this initiative. Resources will be available on the HHS Web site in addition to the USDA Center for Nutrition Policy and Promotion's forthcoming interactive tool, allowing users to track and assess their diet and physical activity.

Who is the author of the ChooseMyPlate.gov material?

Everything on the ChooseMyPlate.gov Web site (Daily Food Plan, Food Tracker, Food Planner, etc.) was developed by a team of nutritionists, dietitians, economists, and policy experts at USDA. The information is based on expert nutrition recommendations for Americans aged 2 years and older from the Dietary Guidelines.

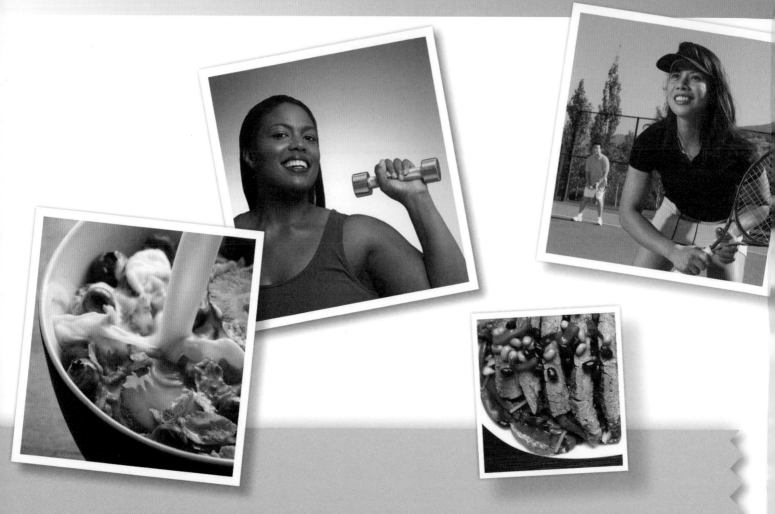

You can find more information about eating healthy and being active at

- http://www.health.gov/dietaryguidelines
- http://www.health.gov/paguidelines
- http://www.healthfinder.gov
- http://www.ChooseMyPlate.gov

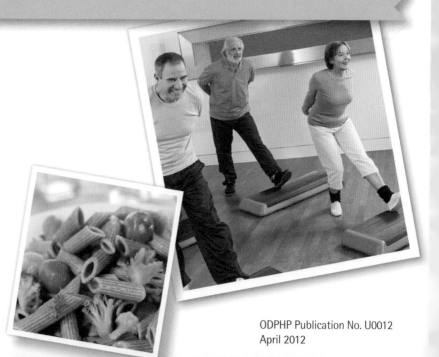

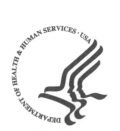

OFFICE OF
DISEASE
PREVENTION AND
HEALTH
PROMOTION

ODPHP Publication No. U0012
April 2012